Life, Almost

www.penguin.co.uk

Life, Almost

*Miscarriage, misconceptions and a search
for answers from the brink of motherhood*

JENNIE AGG

torva

TRANSWORLD PUBLISHERS
Penguin Random House, One Embassy Gardens,
8 Viaduct Gardens, London sw11 7bw
www.penguin.co.uk

Transworld is part of the Penguin Random House group of companies
whose addresses can be found at global.penguinrandomhouse.com

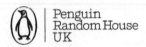

First published in Great Britain in 2023 by Torva
an imprint of Transworld Publishers

The extract on p. vii is from W. Szymborska, *Map: Collected and Last Poems*
(London, HarperCollins, 2016).
The extract on p. 283 from 'East Coker', from *Four Quartets* by T. S. Eliot,
reproduced by permission of Faber & Faber.

A CIP catalogue record for this book
is available from the British Library.

ISBN 9781911709046

Typeset in 13/15.5pt Bembo by Jouve (UK), Milton Keynes
Printed and bound in Great Britain by Clays Ltd, Elcograf S.p.A.

The authorized representative in the EEA is Penguin Random House Ireland,
Morrison Chambers, 32 Nassau Street, Dublin D02 YH68.

Penguin Random House is committed to a sustainable future
for our business, our readers and our planet. This book is made
from Forest Stewardship Council® certified paper.

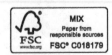

For all the 'almosts'.
Mine – and yours.

'*So you're here? Still dizzy from another dodge,*
close shave, reprieve?
One hole in the net and you slipped through?
I couldn't be more shocked or speechless.
Listen,
how your heart pounds inside me.'

Wisława Szymborska, 'Could Have'

'*We learn geology the morning after the earthquake.*'

Ralph Waldo Emerson, *The Conduct of Life*

Contents

Prologue

'You can't be a little bit pregnant'

(October 2019 – pregnant?)

I hold the pregnancy test up, trying to get a clearer view. I'm studying it with all the intensity of a laboratory scientist, or perhaps a collector examining a new, rare specimen they've trapped between plates of glass. The light in our bathroom is pale and cold, flattened by the beige wall tiles I did not choose. I tilt the test slowly back and forth; this way, then that. I have waited the required ten minutes with practised patience. I have precisely – expertly – saturated the test strip with my own urine. I have dutifully read and reread the instruction leaflet even though, in truth, I more than know the drill by now.

Come on, tell me I'm pregnant.

I have been pregnant enough times to strongly suspect that I am this time, too. There have been signs – signs that only someone who has been trying for a baby for the best part of four years would bother to notice. A furtive heaviness to my breasts. Slight, needling pains deep in my pelvis a little over a week ago. The ghost of a feeling a little like jet lag – a not-quite nausea.

Nothing so crudely blatant as full-on morning sickness (as the movies would have you believe is always the first clue a woman is expecting). No. It's more like a premonition. A sense of one's cells realigning, shifting some inner equilibrium you didn't know you had until it's been knocked off-kilter. I know this feeling so well. A nervous, fluttery excitement, somewhere between physical and emotional. As delicate as a moth's wings – and just as easily squashed.

'Not Pregnant.'

The read-out on the digital fertility monitor on the floor in front of me is unequivocal. But I remain unconvinced, certain in what and how I feel. I know enough by now to know that these things are infinitely more complicated.

It's sometimes said that 'you can't be a little bit pregnant'. It seems harmlessly and unquestionably true, doesn't it? I used to believe it myself. You are either pregnant or you aren't; there can be no in-between. As an expression, it's intended to demonstrate that a given scenario is either/or; black or white. The assumption is that pregnancy is the ultimate binary experience. The implication is that only a very stupid person would believe themselves to be 'a little bit pregnant'. There's either a second line on a pregnancy test, or there isn't. If you're pregnant, you'll have a baby in nine months. If you're not, you won't. That's the stark dividing line drawn in the collective consciousness.

With all due respect to the collective consciousness, it's wrong.

As I have come to know all too well, pregnancy has many, blurry shades of grey. There are all sorts of ways you could, in fact, consider yourself to be 'a little bit pregnant'. From a so-called 'chemical' pregnancy (a very early miscarriage, after a pregnancy test has proven positive, but before the pregnancy has progressed enough to be visible on an ultrasound scan) to a 'missed' miscarriage (when the embryo or foetus dies, but a woman's body doesn't register the loss, there are no symptoms of miscarriage such as pain or bleeding, and pregnancy hormones remain high, meaning you may still *feel* pregnant). Then there's molar pregnancy, when something goes awry in the fertilizing of an egg so that rather than a baby and placenta a mass of abnormal cells develops and burrows into the womb lining. Or an ectopic pregnancy, where an embryo grows in the cramped, impossible space inside a fallopian tube or in another place outside of the womb. In all of these instances, you are not going to have a baby, but you are not *not* pregnant, either. You are both. You are neither.

Alternatively, you can simply be pregnant, but your body hasn't yet made enough of the pregnancy hormone, HCG, for a test to be able to confirm it. Sometimes, the line between pregnant or not – life or not – is so fine it's literally invisible.

Knowing this is why, on a sunless morning in the week the clocks go back, I'm sitting in my bathroom, knickers around my ankles, squinting hard at a pregnancy-test strip long after I should have accepted the result and got on with my day. No newcomer to the conception game, I have been using a comprehensive bit of fertility kit that involves testing your urine every single day of your menstrual cycle – first to detect the hormones that precipitate ovulation and then, later, to spot rising levels of HCG (human chorionic gonadotropin). The test strips are inserted into a little machine with a digital display, which interprets the chemistry for you. With answers given in plain English, rather than crosses or stripes of dye, it's supposed to remove the element of doubt – the second-guessing. Even so, I've still ended up ejecting the strip from the monitor to see the raw data for myself, wondering if there is in fact a hint of a second 'pink for pregnant' line next to the control line, just barely visible to the naked eye, but which is still too faint for the monitor's sensor to register.

A shadow of a positive pregnancy result like this has its own nickname in fertility circles and online chatrooms: a 'squinter'. A squat, ugly word to contain such fragile hope. I inch the strip closer to the window behind me, hoping that a squinter is what I'm looking at here. Sometimes I think I see a gleam of palest pink – a drop of blood in milk – only for the test to look unyieldingly paper-white the next second. Now you see me, now you don't.

I put the test back on the floor and take a picture of it on my phone in case that somehow makes the contrast plainer to see. It doesn't.

If I sound desperate, it's because I am. I need to know with an urgency that goes beyond the usual monthly frustration that will be familiar to anyone who has had to put a bit of effort into getting pregnant. It's a cycle in which your world truncates into two-week blocks: the first half of the month dedicated to pinpointing ovulation and timing sex accordingly, then the second half to waiting until you can take a pregnancy test or for your period to arrive. For approximately ten to fourteen days, it can feel as though everything hinges on the answer to one question. 'Am I pregnant?' From what your life will look like next year to whether you can have a guilt-free glass of wine of an evening. Living with this kind of tunnel vision is infuriating enough in the best of circumstances, but in my case the desperation runs deeper because a positive pregnancy test will not be the end of uncertainty, only the beginning. After four previous miscarriages, for me, and for my husband Dan, the tunnel seems so much longer and darker. The reason I so badly want to know if I am pregnant right now is because, if I am, I know it could well be for the last time, whatever happens. I don't know how much more of this we have left in us. I don't know if I can put us through it all again.

There are still two days until my period is due. This, I know, is soon enough for a sensitive test to reliably detect a pregnancy, but I also know that there's still time for a test that appears negative today to be followed up by a decisively positive one in forty-eight hours' time. Essentially, for all of my efforts this morning, I am none the wiser. It could still go either way. And I've been sitting in the bathroom so long, my foot has gone to sleep.

Reluctantly, I pack away the fertility monitor with its pipettes and plastic sample pots. I delete the picture of the test strip from my phone, so I am not tempted to keep staring at it all day. I wait two days before I test again, an act of self-discipline that feels superhuman. This time, I test using the fertility monitor and also with a separate shop-bought test; just to be sure, I choose one that promises accurate results from six days before your period is due. This time, the second pink line that appears is undeniable. I watch it assert itself as liquid seeps through the weft of the shop-bought test strip. Happiness balloons inside me, along with the satisfaction of being proved right. At the same time, fear crawls up into my throat and lodges there, indefinitely, impossible to ignore or swallow back down.

I have my answer, at last, and the monitor confirms it in writing: Pregnant. I am pregnant, for a fifth time. The much, much bigger question is how long I will stay that way.

Introduction

What we mean when we talk about miscarriage

Something I was told when training to be a journalist was that the really big stories find people even if they're not reading or watching the news. In October 2020, almost a year to the day after I discovered I was pregnant for the fifth time, news broke that the model, author, and TV personality Chrissy Teigen had miscarried her baby boy Jack – her third child with her husband, the singer John Legend – halfway through the pregnancy. I was hiding out at my mum's house at the time, exhausted and overwhelmed, feeling a bit sorry for myself, and spending a week unplugged from my laptop and social media accounts, without my usual newspaper subscriptions and radio alarm tuned to the *Today* programme. The news found me anyway. An editor friend texted me to ask if I'd write about it for her.

Teigen had shared the news of their loss via her Instagram page. 'We are shocked and in the kind of deep pain you only hear about, the kind of pain we've never felt before,' she wrote, alongside a series of black and white photographs taken at the hospital. The pictures are devastatingly intimate. In one, an epidural is about to be administered into Teigen's back. In another, she leans forward on the trolley-bed, hands clasped as if in prayer, eyes down. In every pained line and shadow of her face, you can read an internal ticker tape that will be familiar to anyone who has had a pregnancy end too soon: Please let them live. *Please.*

In several other, later images, Teigen and her husband cradle their baby boy, his face obscured inside a standard-issue hospital blanket. Their expressions could be those of any other new parents, that complicated mixture of primal love, intense pride, and plain old exhaustion. Only the bundle in their arms tells the whole story: too small, too soon.

The close-quarters emotion of these pictures proved too much for some. Opinions simmered, both below the line and from media commentators, debating whether there was something wrong about sharing this moment. Criticism ranged from mild concern over a grieving couple's state of mind, and a feeling that some things are best kept private, to culture-war cruelty, such as the US congressional candidate who declared in a tweet (since deleted) that he hoped Teigen – who is vocally pro-choice – would 'reevaluate [her] thoughts on abortion after their heartbreaking experience. It's not a clump of cells. It's either a baby or it's not.'[1] (In fact, Teigen would later go on to say that she eventually came to understand what happened as a termination rather than a miscarriage, as labour had been induced to save her life, even though her son would not survive.) Yet, for many, many others, Teigen's post acted as a relief valve, allowing their own stories of miscarriage to pour out. At the time of writing, her Instagram post has been 'liked' 11.4 million times. There are more than half a million comments underneath it, many from women sharing the details and memories of their own lost pregnancies. In the ensuing media coverage, the same word came up again and again: 'taboo'. '*Could Chrissy Teigen's courage break the baby loss taboo?*' '*Miscarriage used to be a taboo, until Chrissy Teigen broke the silence.*'

Miscarriage is almost always framed this way: a silent problem that can be fixed by talking about it. '*Why we need to talk about miscarriage*', headlines entice. Articles reference the 'secret pain' and 'stigma'. When someone shares their story publicly, they are 'speaking out' and 'opening up'; we talk of bravery and breaking the silence. I've done it myself. I've written those headlines and I've had them written about me when I've shared my own experiences. It's a media cycle that feels increasingly familiar. In 2018, two years before Teigen made her heartbreaking announcement, the same phrases circulated after former First Lady Michelle Obama spoke of how 'lost and alone' she felt after the miscarriage she'd had before her children were born: '*Michelle Obama opens up*'; '*Michelle Obama reveals she had a miscarriage in effort to end stigma*'. And the same sorts of words echoed across the internet once more when Meghan, Duchess of Sussex, wrote movingly for the *New York Times* about miscarrying what would have been her second child – a revelation that came less than two months after Teigen's: '*Miscarriage is still a taboo*'; '*The Duchess of Sussex shares her "unbearable grief" of miscarriage – and breaks down a taboo*'. Every time there is a story like this, other women's stories come flooding in. Journalists – like me – are commissioned for the features pages in the days following the original news story. Comments sections fill up with condolences and stories offered up in solidarity. With this in mind, I understand why an impression would solidify of a taboo that is being steadily dismantled.

But is it? Any discussion tends to be fleeting and incomplete. There is, perhaps, an illusion of increasing openness that doesn't match up to the way miscarriage is actually experienced. Stories of miscarriage tend to be told only in certain spaces, from a certain angle, from certain kinds of people. What's more, talking about miscarriage is often presented as a self-contained solution, rather than one small part in bringing about actual improvements to medical care or any deeper, scientific understanding of this part of the human experience.

Widely publicized stories, like Meghan's, Chrissy's and

Michelle's, may well give other women leave to speak about miscarriage in a way they feel they can't normally – and yet it seems a transient sort of permission. For a start, it would be wrong to assume that media stories about miscarriage are a recent development. Newspaper reports on the miscarriages of public figures (or, often, the wives of public figures) can be traced back at least as far as the 1930s. Miscarriage was also a popular topic for health periodicals in the 1940s and '50s. Articles drawing on the experiences of non-celebrity women, which frame miscarriage as a silent, unrecognized kind of grief, started appearing in women's magazines back in the 1980s – the decade I was born.

And yet, from news cycle to news cycle, from one high-profile miscarriage to the next, the appetite and gratitude for these stories from others who have experienced miscarriage doesn't seem to diminish. What's clear to me is that there is an unmet need here that runs much deeper; that there are structural, cultural, and medical barriers that are not being dismantled – however much the word 'miscarriage' appears in headlines. How is it that miscarriage has been written about my entire life and yet, when it happened to me, I was largely clueless? How can it be all around us – and simultaneously nowhere to be seen?

I'd heard of miscarriage before I had one; of course I had, and the reality is that most people have heard of miscarriage and they know, in the broadest sense, what it means. 'Miscarriage': it's a word that seems designed to be spoken out of the side of the mouth. Hurried; hushed. It practically begs for the conversation to be over almost as soon as it has begun. Knowing about the hypothetical possibility of miscarriage is why Dan and I were waiting to tell people about our first pregnancy until after twelve weeks, in case 'something' happened. In this way, the threat of miscarriage is built into the very foundations of the modern pregnancy experience. And yet it remains a tenuous half-thought. For some reason, you don't really believe it will happen to you . . . until it does.

The gulf between what I knew about miscarriage and what it was actually like to go through went beyond the usual gap between knowledge and experience. When I miscarried the first time, I had a completely skewed sense of how likely it was to happen to me. I had very little idea what a miscarriage would actually be like, look like, hurt like. I had no notion of how deeply it would affect me. Neither was I prepared for the fact that it could, and would, happen again and again, with no medical explanation forthcoming. I also had no idea that having four miscarriages would push me to the brink; that it would take me to a place where I wasn't certain life was worth living any more and that, in turn, it would force me to live in a different way.

Of course, I could never have known the full extent to which miscarriage would uproot my life, or how it would permanently fracture my relationship with pregnancy, any more than any of us can predict the future. But I should have been much, much better prepared. Because, on top of being a university-educated woman, living in a wealthy country with universal healthcare, I am also a health journalist. For quite a while after my first miscarriage, this made me feel ashamed: ashamed that as a professional who is supposed to know about common conditions affecting the human body, I knew so little about pregnancy loss. I didn't know what a 'missed' miscarriage was. I didn't know that sometimes you had to have surgery after a miscarriage. I didn't know what to do with the tiny body that came out of me. I didn't know that it's estimated that almost one in five women are afflicted with PTSD-like symptoms after an early miscarriage (defined as a miscarriage that happens before thirteen weeks, the end of the first trimester). I didn't know that, for people who lose pregnancy after pregnancy, there is currently no known treatment with high-quality evidence that shows it can help. And it was only after my third miscarriage that I discovered that no official record is kept of how many miscarriages happen each year. Perhaps you didn't know these things either. Perhaps you, like me, only learned them through painful, personal experience. But I have come to see that this not knowing was not a failing on my part – not personally and not professionally. This is a collective failing.

In spring 2021, an editorial in one of the world's oldest and most respected medical journals, the *Lancet*, called for worldwide reform of miscarriage care. 'For too long miscarriage has been minimised and often dismissed,' it admonished. 'The lack of medical progress should be shocking. Instead, there is a pervasive acceptance.' There are an estimated 23 million miscarriages globally every year. That works out at around 44 per minute – 44 pregnancies that will have ended in the time it takes you to read to the end of this paragraph. As many as one in four will lose a pregnancy in their lifetime. An estimated one in twenty will go through it more than once. How can an experience that affects so many still be so profoundly misunderstood? This book is my attempt to answer that question. Through my own experience, and through conversations with experts – from gynaecologists and embryologists to psychologists and anthropologists – I will uncover the many things we get wrong about miscarriage, all the things we have yet to learn, and the scientific and social questions we have yet even to ask. I will try to explain both how we got here and why we tolerate the status quo. More than that, I hope to convince you that this simply isn't good enough. Not only is it inhumane, undermining what can be a defining and traumatic experience in the lives of millions, it's outdated, unscientific, and more than a little bit sexist. Why do we expect people to just put up and shut up? Why do we tolerate such a seismic gap in our understanding of how women's bodies work? Beyond that, how can we be so uninterested, so blasé, about the origins of human life?

An interesting piece of research published in 2020 that sought to examine the general public's knowledge of miscarriage found that while 83 per cent of the people the researchers interviewed knew someone who'd experienced a miscarriage, just over one third had actually discussed it with a family member or friend.[2] They also found that 61 per cent of people underestimated how common miscarriage is, with only 28 per cent correctly identifying that between one in five and one in six pregnancies end this way. Men were three times more likely than women to underestimate how often miscarriages happen, as were those without children. A 2015 survey by Tommy's, the pregnancy- and baby-loss charity, found that out of more than 6,000 women, two thirds felt they couldn't even talk to their best friend about their miscarriage.[3] There is evidently a gulf between the public conversation around miscarriage and the private, lived experience that doesn't seem to have narrowed, regardless of however many women have 'come forward'. Chrissy Teigen, the Duchess of Sussex, and Michelle Obama join a long line of famous women who have spoken about losing a pregnancy: Beyoncé, Courteney Cox, Mariah Carey, Sharon Stone, Nicole Kidman, Alanis Morissette, Pink, Gwyneth Paltrow, Lily Allen … ('Celebrity miscarriage', it turns out, is the kind of desperate thing you google in the small, sad hours of the night.)

Two of Hollywood's most iconic women, Marilyn Monroe and Audrey Hepburn, endured miscarriages in the full glare of the public eye – as did Debbie Reynolds, Elizabeth Taylor, and Sophia Loren. The first of Jackie Kennedy's five pregnancies ended in a miscarriage at the three-month mark – a fact that was known and widely reported once she became First Lady. Yoko Ono and Marianne Faithfull endured the indignity of having their pregnancy losses – in the same week in 1968 – reduced to a single newspaper story, lumped together in the copy by dint of their status as rock 'n' roll 'girlfriends'.

In 2016, the Queen's granddaughter Zara Tindall released a statement saying she had lost the baby she'd been expecting – the pregnancy having been publicly announced less than a month previously. Before that, in 2001, Sophie, Countess of

Wessex, who is married to the Queen's youngest son, Edward, had an ectopic pregnancy. Standing outside the London hospital where his wife was being treated, Prince Edward told reporters of their 'traumatic experience'. Less than a year later, it was widely reported that the barrister Cherie Booth, whose husband Tony Blair was then the UK prime minister, had miscarried – in fact, she fielded questions from the media shortly after undergoing surgery to remove the pregnancy.

In popular culture, miscarriage has made storylines in everything from *Sex and the City* to *The Archers*. There are miscarriage plots in TV's *Desperate Housewives* (2005), *Game of Thrones* (2011), *Gossip Girl* (2012), *Grey's Anatomy* (2019), *King of Queens* (2001), *Six Feet Under* (2005), *This Is Us* (2017), and *Veep* (2012). It crops up in glossy, quality dramas (*Mad Men*, 2013) and in reality TV (*Selling Sunset*, 2019; *Married at First Sight UK*, 2021; *The Real Housewives of Salt Lake City*, 2021). Sometimes its portrayal is sensitive and probing, while in other instances it's little more than a plot device.

In fiction, miscarriage features in blockbuster novels – such as *The Time Traveler's Wife* (2003), *The Help* (2009), and *The Light Between Oceans* (2012) – and in their subsequent film adaptations. It's the subject of the Ed Sheeran song 'Small Bump' (2012) and of 'More' (2020) by Generation Z pop star Halsey, who has spoken about miscarrying in the middle of one of their concerts. It's been written about by female journalists, memoirists and novelists, from Caitlin Moran and Ariel Levy to Maggie O'Farrell and Candice Carty-Williams. Miscarriage crops up – pun fully intended – in Jilly Cooper's *The Man Who Made Husbands Jealous* (1993). Even the formidable and famously unsentimental Diana Athill recounted a miscarriage she'd had forty years previously, which nearly killed her, in an essay for the literary magazine *Granta* in 2010. While the account would later be included in a volume of her memoirs, when the piece was originally published it was written – unusually – in the third person, keeping the reader one step removed, not quite acknowledging that this was, in fact, Athill's own experience.

You can go back further and further and still find miscarriage, hiding in plain sight, in the artistic output of women. Sylvia Plath's 1961 poem 'Parliament Hill Fields' summarizes the invisible grief after a miscarriage that will be familiar to many: 'Your absence is inconspicuous; Nobody can tell what I lack.' Almost a century ago now, Frida Kahlo captured both the livid violence of miscarriage and the sterile emptiness you feel afterwards. In her painting *Henry Ford Hospital* (1932), blood spills across a white sheet, a foetus the colour of a bruise unspooling on its umbilical thread away from Frida the would-be mother, as it floats against an indifferent blue sky.

Today, there are countless personal blogs and social media pages dedicated to documenting the experience of pregnancy loss (my own website and social media feeds included). In particular, the explosion in popularity of Instagram, podcasts, and email newsletters, which all confer a kind of intimacy and are less easily interrupted than other mediums, seems to have led to ever more open discussions, especially between women. Most recently, the video-sharing app TikTok has offered a new, succinct – and often enjoyably snarky – way to sum up aspects of this experience, such as the unhelpful things people say to you afterwards. And yet we shouldn't mistake any of this for evidence of a job done – that we have a firm grasp on what miscarriage is like or why it happens.

For all that miscarriage is 'out there', people continue to say the same things when they experience it for themselves. With not a little irony, miscarriage is, by all accounts, profoundly isolating. It is 'lonely, painful and demoralizing almost on a cellular level' in the words of Michelle Obama. The Duchess of Sussex suggested that we seem to be trapped in 'a cycle of solitary mourning'. Why? There are more than twenty years between Michelle Obama's experience of miscarriage and

Meghan's and yet they echo each so closely. Why has so little improved for us? Why do women continue to live in the 'silence after silence' that Plath described in her poem more than sixty years ago? Why are we still caught unawares by the depth of emotion – of love – that can accompany early pregnancy; 'that someone who didn't yet exist could have the power to create spring', as Diana Athill puts it? Why, for that matter, has there been so little medical progress in understanding what causes miscarriages? And why – to ask a really wild question – do we just accept that so many miscarriages still happen in the first place? Why don't we know how to prevent them? In short, what are we *not* talking about when we talk about miscarriage?

If miscarriage is not a taboo in the truest sense – literally unspeakable, unheard of – what it *is* is profoundly misunderstood, under-researched, and under-acknowledged. The danger, if we keep labelling it a taboo without digging much deeper, is that there'll be a backlash before anything improves materially for those miscarriage affects. We risk straightforward sympathy starting to feel stale to jaded palates. There is a damning eye-roll of a line sometimes deployed in response to someone sharing their experience of pregnancy or new motherhood: 'She thinks she's the first woman ever to have a baby.' How long before the same knee-jerk, get-over-yourself-luv misogyny is the latest Hot Take when it comes to pregnancy loss, too? How far are we from some unfathomably unkind columnist snipe-typing 'You'd think she's the first woman to have a miscarriage' the next time someone in the public eye shares their grief for a baby they never got to bring home?

Actually, it's possible this moment has already arrived. In response to Meghan's *New York Times* piece in 2020, the website Spiked ran a sneering op-ed headlined '*Do we really need to know about Meghan Markle's miscarriage?*'[4] On Twitter, trolls targeted the journalist and author Elizabeth Day – who has written about her own miscarriages and desire to be a mother – after she praised Meghan and Chrissy Teigen for 'speaking openly about something that historically has given women so much pain, shame and trauma'. Dismissive replies to Day's tweet (some since deleted) accused both Chrissy and Meghan of attention-seeking and narcissism, meanwhile Day herself was told that she'd know how common it was for women to share such stories, if only she had children. And one Sunday-newspaper columnist criticized Meghan's account of miscarriage as 'strangely glossy and idealised' in a piece headlined '*Can we stop all the woe-is-me over our wombs? We're women, not victims*'.[5] I've had a taste of this sort of compassion fatigue myself. A piece I'd written for a newspaper, days after my fourth miscarriage, was pulled at the last minute after a (male) editor had demurred that 'Oh, loads of women have miscarriages.' He made this objection to a colleague, rather than to my face, but it still feels like a gut-punch, even now.

Yes, you know intellectually that you are not the first woman ever to have had a miscarriage, but the point is that you are made to *feel* as though you might be. And as with the realities of pregnancy and childbirth, if women describe their experience of losing a baby in ways that feel familiar to an older generation, that should give us pause to reflect rather than dismiss it as unoriginal and therefore unworthy of examination. If women continue to express shock, pain, and loneliness in response to what is widely acknowledged to be commonplace, that should be a red-light warning that something's wrong with the system. It suggests that our lived experience is chafing against the constructs placed around it; that there is a gap between what people feel and need after a miscarriage and what society allows for. Like couples whose arguments over dropped socks and other minor transgressions escalate and circle back, eventually reopening the old wounds of a decade's worth of fights, what we are really saying – what we really mean when we call miscarriage a taboo – is: nothing has changed. *You're not listening to me.*

Because, for all the media stories and the conversations it supposedly generates, we have yet to make proper sense of miscarriage – both in terms of the biology and its true impact on people who have one. We have not metabolized it and assimilated it into social norms and modern culture. The convention is still to hide a pregnancy until the end of the first trimester, which these days can be a full two months after someone finds out they're pregnant. For all it may seem miscarriage is 'out in the open' and increasingly talked about, it is not routinely written into HR policies, people still don't know what to say to their friends who endure it (if they know about a loss in the first place), and scientific research, tests, and treatments for those who endure multiple miscarriages are thin on the ground. As a subject, it is still obscured by myths, medical mysteries, and misconceptions, all of which have been permitted to go unchallenged thanks to age-old squeamishness and shame around women's bodies, and our collective ineloquence on matters of grief. The bloody, untimely end of a pregnancy sits at the centre of a perfect Venn diagram of things that make us uncomfortable: sex, death and periods.

In the ABC interview in which she disclosed her experience of both miscarriage and infertility, Michelle Obama memorably said that 'it's the worst thing that we do to each other as women, not share the truth about our bodies and how they work – and how they don't work'.[6] I agree. But I also think this isn't only about what women do or do not choose to say. There's something deeper going on here – something more than can be fixed by individual acts of disclosure, however courageous and honest. If you ask me, the worst thing we do to women *as a society* is to not believe them when they tell us about the things that happen to their bodies. Women have been trying to talk about miscarriage and to change the discourse around it for years. We just haven't been paying enough attention.

1

'It's so common'

(November 2019 — 6 weeks pregnant)

Apart from telling Dan that I am, in fact, pregnant again, we do not discuss it any more than is necessary. We are neither of us ready to look it in the eye yet. If we have to mention it at all, we only allude to it, signalling our conjoined fear and hope through nods, half-glances, and brisk hand-squeezes. Any sentence about the pregnancy almost always begins 'If', never 'When'. If this, then that. If that, then this. *If, if, if* . . .

For the first week of the pregnancy, I do precisely nothing about it. When seven days are up, I allow myself to take another test, a digital one, which will estimate how many weeks along I am. As has become something of a ritual, I send Dan a photo of the positive test stick.

'Whose is it?' he replies.

It wasn't really funny the first time, but there is something comforting about the recurring joke — a tiny fragment of us salvaged from before, when pregnancy still felt normal. Easy. Even fun.

To be pregnant again after previous miscarriages is to live –
very consciously – at the fork of two alternative lives. You try
to think as little as possible about what's going on inside your
body, while, of course, thinking about it all the time. Alive or
dead? Baby or miscarriage? In every possible scenario, you plan
for the two outcomes. To a certain extent, you are forced to
buy into both possibilities simultaneously. You cannot truly
believe it will work out, but you have to proceed as though you
are pregnant anyway, until a scan proves otherwise. Alive *and*
dead. Schrödinger's foetus.

You treat yourself as your own personal research study: a
sample of one. Perhaps you take a different brand of prenatal
vitamin this time. Or you do different exercise. You do no
exercise at all. You drink less caffeine. You drink no caffeine at
all. You are more careful. Or you are less careful, because you've
been unimpeachably careful before and look at where it got
you. Mostly, though, you just wait.

I don't phone our GP. Because I know that if I do, they will
want me to make an appointment to 'book in' for antenatal care,
setting in motion a chain of appointments and scans I might only
have to cancel again in a few weeks. I've attended such appointments before, only to find out shortly after that the baby has
died – indeed, in all likelihood, was already dead as I filled in
forms with a cheerful midwife. I also do not start browsing for
baby clothes or maternity dresses. In the event of another miscarriage, I do not want to scent a trail for adverts that will stalk me
across the internet long after googling 'bleeding eight weeks
pregnant' – a red flag that internet company algorithms are apparently oblivious to. Instead, I bury myself in work, ignoring the
familiar fatigue that begins wrapping itself around my muscles
and slowing the connection speed of my brain. Yet I continue to
keep score, turning over the numbers in my mind as if updating a
site-safety card for my own body: Five days without incident . . .
Six days without incident . . . Ten days without incident.

When I need something to take the edge off, I do another pregnancy test and try to take heart in the stripes of dye that are darker and more confident than they were the last time I tested. When the end of one week ticks over into the next, I search for comfort in the window of another digital test, which confirms that 'Pregnant 1–2 weeks' has turned into 'Pregnant 2–3 weeks' and then 'Pregnant 3 weeks+'. A knot of something akin to determination tightens each time; a feeling that a small hurdle has been cleared – although I also know these tiny achievements could still amount to nothing.

The clenched holding pattern Dan and I now find ourselves in is so unlike the first time we found out we were expecting. And yet the dates of this fifth pregnancy mirror that first one so closely, it's unnerving. I found out about both in mid-autumn, which means a July due date. Not that I look up the exact date this time, using an online calculator. I don't need to. The maths is still imprinted. And this time there will be no dates for the diary. No names. No using the word 'baby'. In this way, what we are experiencing is a shadow pregnancy – the dark twin of our first.

Back then, all I'd felt had been an uncomplicated joy. I was simply thrilled to be pregnant, after ten months of trying. Not an unusually long time, but longer than I'd expected. That time, now three years ago, the knowledge that we were going to start a family was a pure golden thread tugging me through the dark, cold months of winter; through furtively sober office parties and a Christmas without Brie or Stilton; through the bone-seeping tiredness and nausea that would loosen its grip on me only in order to let a primal, carnivorous hunger take its turn. For weeks, I felt awful – and I didn't mind. Pregnancy could have me. That glimmer of secret knowledge was stitched in tight. I wanted this. I was ready for this. I *loved* this.

That first time, I wasted no time in putting together an inventory of everything we would need for our new life. The morning after I proudly showed Dan our first positive pregnancy test, I stayed propped up in bed, receiving cups of tea and rounds of toast, roaming the internet on my phone in search of pram recommendations and aspirational nursery designs. By the end of the first week, I had a carefully selected arsenal of books sitting in my Amazon basket, ready to be ordered the minute we got home from the twelve-week scan. Because, for all my giddy excitement, there was still this superstitious hesitation. I never thought to question the feeling that it would be 'bad luck' to actually buy anything yet, or where that impression came from. Dan and I had tacitly agreed we wouldn't share our news 'in case anything happened', without truly believing that anything would. As far as we knew, it almost never did.

We were blissfully naive. We talked about names for our baby a lot, back then. Dan would suggest names of Newcastle United players, which I'd veto. I'd suggest names of Forties starlets or something fashionably Scandinavian-sounding, which he'd veto. Day-to-day, we kept up a steady patter about the kind of parents we wanted to be, rehearsing our ideas and convincing ourselves that we could break the mould we'd seen slowly forming around us, cast by friends who'd already started their families. First of all, it wasn't going to change us. Definitely not. We were still going to be able to talk about something that wasn't Peppa Pig. We would do our best to keep on top of who was in the shadow cabinet and which restaurant was *the* place to queue for food in London. And we wouldn't be buying the endless plastic tat that everyone else we knew with children seemed to accumulate. We told ourselves these things, believing them earnestly, but also knowing deep down that we didn't mind becoming just like everyone else. That was, after all, part of the joy: that it was our turn for that life-changing, devouring kind of love.

On New Year's Eve that year, Dan had to wake me at midnight. By then, I was ten weeks pregnant. I'd been in bed since

10.30 p.m., I was exhausted, and I was very, very sober. But, at thirty years old, it was the best New Year's Eve I'd ever had. We'd chosen to stay in: just us. I'd made us dinner: beef, slow-cooked in the oven in a bright-orange pot, the meat falling off the bone, rich in iron and umami. We went through the motions of choosing a film to watch, although we both knew I would fall asleep on the sofa shortly after the opening credits. I don't remember what we picked. I don't remember going up to bed, but I do remember how Dan kissed me when he woke me at midnight – once on the mouth, and once on the stomach. One for me, one for the baby we believed would be born that year.

'You can go back to sleep now,' he said.

Pride and expectation prickled across my skin. I'd drifted off, hand curled around my miniature bump, half-listening to the fizz and pop of fireworks at unseen parties. The whole sky over our sleepy, commuter-belt town was exploding in celebration of this brilliant thing that was about to happen to us.

The difference between pregnancy before and after miscarriage is rarely acknowledged by the world at large or, indeed, by the antenatal system you have no choice but to engage with. There's a curious doublethink expected of you in the early stages of any pregnancy. On the one hand the convention is to keep the pregnancy a secret until the end of the first trimester, when the risk of miscarriage is thought to recede, a practice that both keeps the true extent of pregnancy loss hidden and also diminishes the status of a pregnancy in its earliest weeks, as if it were in some way less real during this time. Yet, simultaneously, everything about modern pregnancy encourages you to invest deeply in your future baby – the 'child in mind', as the psychotherapist Julia Bueno has astutely labelled it.[1] Pregnancy apps do not start from twelve weeks, they start from the moment you get a positive test result, sometimes even earlier. 'This week your baby is the size of a poppy seed!' they tell you excitedly. You're advised to take folic acid for the benefit of the baby from the get-go (indeed, both the NHS and the American Pregnancy Association recommend that you take it as soon as you start trying to conceive). You are booked in for scans many weeks ahead. In their chapters on the first trimester, pregnancy books say cutesy things like 'Take a good look at your waist: it may be the last time you'll see it for a while' and make suggestions such as starting a bump photo-diary, even if there's not much bump yet to photograph ('Lights, camera . . . baby!' chirrups one ubiquitous handbook). Even the more muted, matter-of-fact advice set out by the NHS in its week-by-week pregnancy guide recommends thinking from week ten about where you might like to give birth, and from week eleven looking into what maternity leave you're legally entitled to. It is easy, therefore, to be lulled into a false sense of security. You may not be broadcasting your news yet, 'just in case', but this is made to feel like a mere formality; a fun tradition, even. It doesn't seem to matter that, with one in four women believed to experience it over the course of their life, miscarriage is 'the commonest complication of pregnancy', as Professor Lesley Regan, head of obstetrics and gynaecology at St Mary's Hospital in London, puts it in her book *Miscarriage: What Every Woman Needs To Know*.[2] Despite the inconvenient statistics, everything around you keeps up a pretence that miscarriage is no more than a remote possibility. It is only once you have to repeat the pregnancy process after a previous loss that the full extent of this illusion – and the emotional gymnastics you are required to perform in its service – becomes truly apparent.

In a pregnancy after a miscarriage, medically you may continue to be referred to as a *primigravida* (a first-timer) whether it's technically your second pregnancy or your seventh. Apart from noting down the details of the previous loss on your antenatal file ('Number of weeks? Any surgery?'), there is little space or time given over to how it might be affecting how you feel about this subsequent pregnancy and how you might wish to approach it. In my third pregnancy, the local antenatal team had wanted me to have my booking-in appointment with them at seven weeks. When I asked if I could possibly wait a bit longer, haltingly explaining my history and the timeline of our last miscarriage – the baby that had, in fact, already been dead when I'd arrived at the first appointment – the woman on the other end of the phone had tutted.

'Thing is,' she sighed, 'it'll make it more difficult for us to get your scan in at the right time, then.' I pictured her staring out of the window, wondering what she was going to have for lunch, while I grappled with the quantum mechanics of this; how I was being expected to worry about a theoretical future scan that I might never need, when my primary concern was whether my pregnancy would survive to the appointment before that. I opened my mouth and then closed it again. Eventually, pleading a packed schedule, I convinced her to push it to what would have been my ninth week – the latest slot they had. There was no baby by then, as it would turn out, and so I had to cancel anyway. But at least I saved us all some paperwork.

Of course, no admin process can accommodate all of life with perfect nuance and sensitivity every time, but miscarriage is far from an exceptional circumstance. Every year, a considerable proportion of those embarking on a pregnancy will previously have lost a baby early on – an estimated 250,000 people, in fact. That's 250,000 of us squashed uncomfortably into a system that essentially pretends miscarriage doesn't happen, won't happen again, and isn't especially relevant to our medical history. In fact, the actual number affected could be even higher. Because here is the first and most fundamental gaping hole in our knowledge around miscarriages – we don't officially know how many happen each year. Not precisely, anyway: the 250,000 figure is a best guess, based on the number of babies born in the UK and what research has shown about the proportion of pregnancies that end in miscarriage,* but, at the time of writing, there is no official record kept. And the UK is far from alone in this. It's a data gap that exists in most countries in the developed world, according to the World Health Organization.[3]

It's something that obstetrician and miscarriage specialist Professor Siobhan Quenby believes needs to change, as the absence of accurate data plays a big part in keeping miscarriage underfunded, understudied, and, ultimately, misunderstood. 'Because we have no data, we have no status,' she tells me. 'The data is not available nationally, and the reasons for that are quite complicated,' she explains. 'It's because some people miscarry

---

* The quoted figure for this also varies significantly. For example, the charity Tommy's concludes that one in four pregnancies end in miscarriage, while the official line from the NHS is that it's one in eight. The US maternity healthcare organization March of Dimes hedges its bets, stating that 10–15 per cent of recognized pregnancies end in miscarriage. In Australia, the government-funded pregnancy advice service states that 'up to 1 in 5 confirmed pregnancies end in miscarriage'. There are several reasons for this inconsistency. Confusion creeps in depending on what countries class as a miscarriage, for a start – in the UK and Ireland it's any pregnancy lost before twenty-four weeks, but in the US and Australia the cut-off point is twenty weeks. The World Health Organization considers it to be twenty-eight weeks. How countries collect and assimilate data on elected abortions also complicates the picture, as it may have a bearing on the true pregnancy rate. Then there are discrepancies as to what is counted as a 'known', 'confirmed' or 'clinically recognized' pregnancy. Miscarriage rates will differ depending on how the data is gathered; for example, miscarriage rates may be higher among women who've had a positive home pregnancy test than among a group of women studied from the time of their first antenatal appointment, as any earlier miscarriages will already have been excluded by default in this latter group. What's more, factors such as how a country's healthcare system is funded can affect how early on women register their pregnancy, which again potentially obscures the true miscarriage rate. For my purposes, I have gone with the estimate that one in five pregnancies end in miscarriage. This is the figure given by the UK's Royal College of Obstetricians and Gynaecologists when looking specifically at early miscarriage – that is, within the first three months of pregnancy. This time-period represents both when the majority of miscarriages are believed to occur and also the boundary of my own experience.

at A&E, some just go to their GP, while others may go to an early-pregnancy unit [EPU]. So, because there are lots of places where you might miscarry, the data is not collected in a complete way. But it doesn't mean it couldn't be.' Currently, even a fairly basic level of information – the number of hospital admissions for miscarriages – is not added to official UK maternity statistics.

This kind of record-keeping shouldn't be seen as mere academic pedantry or a 'nice-to-have'. Miscarriage rates could (and should) be considered a vital marker of public health. For her part, Professor Quenby believes that hospital trusts should be required to report their area's miscarriage rate in the same way they are required to report their rates of stillbirth and neonatal death. Both of these are known to rise where there are high levels of social deprivation, for example, and it's likely that miscarriage rates do, too. Therefore 'it needs to be something we care about, socially', she says. 'The miscarriage rate is a public health measure. Things like poor medical care, poorly controlled diabetes, obesity, and high levels of pollution all inform miscarriage rates. It's really serious.'

What's more, without properly reported, comprehensive miscarriage data it's harder to understand whether different groups are being disproportionately affected – and, if so, why. It's only recently been reported that Black women have a higher risk of miscarriage than white women – as much as 40 per cent higher, according to research published in the *Lancet* in 2021.[4] It is further evidence of the scandalous racial inequalities that exist when it comes to maternity care. Yet we only know this about miscarriage because of a few studies – not from any sort of official record-keeping. Owing to data that is routinely collected and analysed in the UK, we now know that Black women have four times the risk of dying during pregnancy or childbirth than white women. *Four times*. While the overall maternal mortality risks are still small in this country, the stark disparity along racial lines is shameful. The same data has also shown up a two-fold difference in the risk of dying for mothers from Asian ethnic backgrounds compared with white mothers.[5] Meanwhile, Black women are twice as likely to have a stillborn baby than white women, while babies born to Asian British women are 60 per cent more likely to die shortly after birth than white babies.[6] What else might we have missed about miscarriage by not bothering to collect the data?

As for socio-economic inequality, women living in the poorest parts of England are significantly more likely to experience stillbirth, pre-term birth, or to have a baby whose growth is severely restricted, according to a 2021 study of more than 1 million births.[7] In fact, the researchers estimated that 24 per cent of stillbirths, 19 per cent of pre-term births and 31 per cent of cases of foetal growth restriction can be attributed to poverty and would not occur if women from the poorest backgrounds had the same risks as the least deprived women. According to Professor Quenby, you would expect to see similar inequalities with miscarriage rates in the UK. 'But without the data, we have no way of knowing for certain,' she says.

We also have no precise way of knowing whether miscarriage rates are improving at all – or getting worse. And when we don't accurately record how many miscarriages happen, it's harder to quantify the wider impact of pregnancy loss, such as the true cost to the health service, the estimated number of mental health days taken as a result of it, or the cost to the economy in terms of lost working days. In 2021, Professor Quenby and a coalition of other leading scientists suggested that the economic cost of miscarriage is at least £471 million per year in the UK.[8] Indeed, they said, the true figure is likely to be even higher, but they were only able to estimate the short-term costs (such as hospital treatment and days off work immediately afterwards) as information on longer-term consequences simply does not exist. And, of course, this absence of cold, hard costs conspires to keep the conversation around miscarriage from being spoken about with conviction to governments, politicians, and big business.

It occurs to me, too, as I wait out the first few weeks of this latest pregnancy, studiously avoiding any contact with the healthcare system, what a vicious cycle we've created. Currently, my fifth pregnancy is flying below the radar. It's as yet unknown to my GP, the local midwife team, or even the specialist clinic where I've been treated since my third miscarriage. If I were to miscarry now, it would be completely untraceable. I wonder how many other pregnancies – and miscarriages – function like this? Hidden from view until it's absolutely necessary to break cover, put off by a healthcare system that doesn't feel designed for us. And yet, the more we go to ground as a coping mechanism, the more the scale of the problem goes unappreciated. No data, no status.

A miscarriage can be graphic in its violence. The first time, two weeks after that blissful New Year's Eve, I woke up one Saturday morning to a warm gush of liquid. Blood. Bright, red blood. I propelled myself out of bed and ran the few metres to our bathroom. I closed the door with one hand, while with the other I tugged my underwear down to half-mast. Immediately, I felt something slide away: something made of blood, but somehow solid at the same time. Someone gave a strangulated sort of scream. Me, I realized a split second later.

'What's happening?' Dan asked from the other side of the wall. 'Jen?'

But I couldn't find the words. I was looking at the bathroom floor. Was this it? Our baby? I couldn't be certain. It didn't look like a baby, only a sad, liver-ish mass. The size of a lime. I stared at it where it lay against the indifferent, grey tile. Perhaps there was still hope. Perhaps this wasn't really it. Perhaps it was still inside, somehow. Although the blood kept on coming.

The bleeding had started the day before, but it had been nothing like this. It had been just a few spots, the colour of rust. At first, I'd told myself it was nothing – I had, after all, had a similar bleed earlier on in the pregnancy that had been just that. We'd gone for an early scan to check and been rewarded with a glimpse of a tiny but insistent six-week heartbeat – little more than a flickering dot on the ultrasound screen; hummingbird-fast but definitely there. *Whump-whump, whump-whump, whump-whump.* I am, I am, I am.

'That's a really good sign,' the midwife had told us. 'Once we've seen a heartbeat, the risk of miscarriage is next to nothing.'

So, more than a month on, I'd tried not to worry about this new bleed too. But, by the afternoon, it was getting worse not better. I'd phoned the GP. It was Friday and I was in the office, at the newspaper where I was working as an editor. At this particular paper, Friday afternoon was just about the worst time in the news cycle you could pick to have a miscarriage. Saturday's paper was the big one, as far as sales were concerned, and the printer's deadline was earlier in the evening than on other days. This meant working with the week's biggest stories in a lot less time. Standards and voices were raised accordingly. The copy was always either too long or too short; too 'chewy' or too bloody obvious. The legal queries and changes would keep coming in a torrent of blue biro, and the eminent 'top expert' who had written something for you would be insisting on approving every comma and caption personally, while also ignoring your chasing emails. Lunch would inevitably be going cold on your desk and the star columnists still wouldn't have filed . . . Hardly the ideal moment to extricate myself so I could walk around the block three times while on hold to the doctor's surgery.

I stood shivering in my shift dress. At just over eleven weeks along, no one knew I was pregnant yet, so I'd left my jacket on the back of my chair in the hope that anyone who needed me would assume I was in the loo, or, better still, a Very Important Meeting. Our GP thought the best thing to do was to come in so they could refer me for a scan – before the surgery closed for the weekend and I was left at the mercy of A&E. I dashed off a quick email to my boss saying I didn't feel well and left before he would have time to read it and ask any questions. This was definitely not how I'd wanted to disclose my pregnancy. As I hurried away down Kensington High Street, I imagined the swivel-chair at my desk three floors up, still spinning in my wake.

The plan was to meet Dan at the surgery. I made the next train in the nick of time and, only once it was pulling safely away from the city, allowed myself to cry. The thought poured through my brain like cold water: *I'm having a miscarriage. And nobody knows.*

The GP's reaction when I arrived was anticlimactically calm.

'I wouldn't worry, it doesn't sound like a lot of blood,' she told us evenly; not unkindly, but perhaps a little bored. (I will come to expect this as the default setting for many doctors, GP receptionists, midwives, and sonographers who find themselves dealing with miscarriage.) She made an appointment for us at our local hospital's early-pregnancy unit for a scan the following morning – 10 a.m., the earliest they could do.

To distract ourselves, Dan and I decided to go out for dinner and to see a film. As we drove to the local multiplex, I was worried, but – whisper it – also a little excited, buoyed by the doctor's reassurances. Our official twelve-week scan was supposed to be happening that coming Tuesday – what would have been our first look at our baby, had it not been for the bleed at six weeks – and I had been counting down the days. I wanted to see my baby again; I wanted that blobby black-and-grey picture to stick on the fridge. Were we about to get a sneak preview? The doctor was right, I told myself, there hadn't been a lot of blood. Not really.

Halfway through dinner, however, that tiny bubble of excitement was skewered by the arrival of cramps – a murmur of the period pain I'd not missed those past three months. And then, there in the bathroom of the Uxbridge branch of Nando's: blood. Fire-engine red, this time. Emergency red. Danger. Stop.

Dan and I watched the film anyway. We'd already bought the tickets and, besides, what else were we going to do? We let it wash over us, willing ourselves to be numbed by the blur of colours and sound. We sat through songs and LA traffic jams. We observed a love scene in an observatory, constellations of stars swimming above us, while a girl in a yellow dress twirled and twirled and twirled.

By the time we went to bed that night, we were fairly certain I was losing the baby – and Google suggested there was nothing any doctor could do if I was. We decided to wait for the 10 a.m. appointment rather than go to A&E that night. Neither of us knew whether this was even the sort of thing you should turn up at Casualty for. Is a miscarriage a medical emergency?* We had no idea. No one had ever told us. It wasn't mentioned in any of the many, many leaflets and pregnancy information sheets I'd been given. But, waking to flooded sheets the next

---

* Although it is distressing, from a medical perspective a miscarriage is not usually a serious threat to health. However, any bleeding – and pain, especially severe abdominal pain or pain in the shoulder-tip, where the shoulder meets the arm – in early pregnancy should be investigated to rule out an ectopic pregnancy, where the embryo grows outside of the uterus (the word ectopic means 'out of place'), usually in the fallopian tube. This can be life-threatening, as the tube can rupture. Medical advice should always be sought for any heavy bleeding – soaking through a sanitary pad in an hour or less – even if you already know it is a confirmed miscarriage and not an ectopic pregnancy. Around one in 100 women who miscarry will experience blood loss severe enough to require a transfusion. There is also a small risk of infection during or after a miscarriage – affecting between one and four women in 100. Signs of infection include a raised temperature, flu-like symptoms and offensive-smelling discharge.

morning, it was obvious waiting was no longer an option. A miscarriage was, evidently, not going to be 'just a heavy period'.

At the hospital's early-pregnancy unit, they send me to A&E because I am bleeding too heavily for them to scan me. Before we'd left home, I'd put in two sanitary pads, but even this is not enough to stop the blood seeping through my thickest jeans and the wool of my winter coat on to the vomit-orange plastic chair in the triage nurse's office. This is where the film reel of my memory stutters and snags. I'm wheeled somewhere, past queues of trolley-beds in corridors. (We're in the middle of a winter flu crisis.) In a side bay, a cannula is stuck in my hand. Somewhere else – before or after, I'm not sure – outside a ward bathroom, a woman shouts at me as the gown I don't remember putting on is gaping open. 'Do you mind?' she barks, flapping her hand at me, and then gestures at her teenage son, who isn't looking at me anyway. She looks so angry, but it doesn't compute. I am trying to get a nurse's attention as I'd gone to the loo and now there is blood on the floor again. Zooming into focus next is Dan's face, his mouth a grim line, as a gynaecologist performs an internal exam on me. When he sees the sharp-beaked speculum, Dan's eyes widen slightly – my stoical, quietly romantic husband, who hates it when I leave the bathroom door even slightly ajar. But he doesn't look away.

Later that afternoon, when the midwife broke the news we knew was coming, she didn't show us the screen. She kept it tactfully tilted from view, in a way I would come to dread, but I caught a glimpse as I got dressed to go home. Black and still. I don't know which was worse: this empty freeze-frame, or the soft, whispery way she said, 'I'm so sorry, Jennifer . . .'

Back at the house, I went straight upstairs to our bedroom, ostensibly to change out of the hospital-issue paper pants. For a while, I just stood, staring, thinking how everything and nothing had changed. Despite moving so far and so fast, we were right back where we started. None of it felt possible. I

could go to the shop now and buy an edition of a newspaper I'd
been working on back when I was still pregnant. I could read
headlines I'd written while still pregnant. Just the day before. I
pictured my desk chair, still spinning, like a roulette wheel, up
on the third floor where I'd left it, really not that long ago.
How many hours had it been since I was still pregnant? How
many minutes?

I thought then of the bottle of folic acid tablets in the kitchen cupboard downstairs, no longer needed. Ditto the day off
I'd booked for the scan and the maternity coat I'd bought in the
sale — too much of a bargain to resist — hanging uselessly at the
back of the wardrobe.

All pointless. All impossible.

In our room, there was no evidence of what had gone on
that morning. It hadn't registered when we'd left for the hospital, but Dan had the presence of mind to strip our bed and
stick the bloodied sheets in the washing machine. No evidence
apart from, I remembered, the thing that may or may not have
been a baby that had fallen on to the bathroom floor. It was still
there, behind the closed door. I scooped it up, wrapped it gently in a shroud of loo paper, and placed it inside the cardboard
box from a recently opened pot of face cream. I left the box on
the bathroom windowsill. Two days later, I flushed it away.

2

'At least it was early'

(November 2019 – 7 weeks pregnant)

Today, Dan and I have an appointment at the recurrent-miscarriage clinic – our first in this fifth pregnancy. The clinic is in central London, so we have to take the train. I know from our previous pregnancy, which was also monitored here for the few weeks it lasted, that they will want to take blood tests and also do an early scan. Is the embryo the right size? Is it in the right place? It's the first hurdle. This morning marks the first point at which we could go from being pregnant to unceremoniously unpregnant, or even some no man's land in between. As we hurtle through subterranean London on a packed rush-hour Tube, I try not to think of the number of ways we could fall at this first fence: an ectopic pregnancy, an anembryonic pregnancy, no visible pregnancy at all . . .

It's been three weeks since I found out I was pregnant for the fifth time, which means I am seven weeks pregnant. Although that does not actually mean I've been pregnant for seven weeks. Not literally. Because pregnancies are dated from the first day

of someone's last period, for the first two weeks or until someone ovulates, there is no pregnancy. The sperm that creates the
embryo that then attaches to the uterus lining has not even
entered the body. Weeks one and two of pregnancy only come
into being retrospectively, around week four, when a home
pregnancy test will be able to detect the hormone HCG. Our
entire framework for pregnancy, then, is built on a foundation
of ambiguity and absence. It causes no end of confusion, not
least among legislators who have sought to reduce abortion
time limits to six weeks, who sometimes mistakenly −
blithely − assume this gives a woman a whole six weeks to
make arrangements, when in fact she only has fourteen days, in
a best-case scenario. At the same time, it obscures the true
parameters of earliest pregnancy. And if someone has a vague
remembrance that for a certain amount of time in what we
label as pregnancy there isn't actually anything there, perhaps
this muddies their understanding of what a miscarriage at five,
six, seven weeks really means. Is this a literal loss of life or only
a hypothetical one?

Even after four very real miscarriages, I am not immune to
this way of thinking. Today, what Dan and I are hoping for −
what we *need* − is a heartbeat. When you are desperate to have a
baby, there is something about that pulsating pinhead of light
on a screen that gives life to the whole endeavour. However cir-
cumspect you are trying to be, it is hard not to imagine this
flash − little more than a quiver − as the point at which it all
begins. This first sighting of a heartbeat can feel like validation.
Proof that this really is the start of something, not just a vague
confabulation of unseen chemicals, hormones and blood. And
yet, while a scan like this may well be the first visible evidence
of life in motion, that's not exactly the same as being the moment
that life begins − an altogether more vexed and complicated
question. The presence of a heartbeat, as Dan and I know only
too well, is also no guarantee that a pregnancy will continue.

A human heartbeat is first detectable on an ultrasound scan between five and a half and six weeks of pregnancy – around three to four weeks after sperm meets egg. A pedant will argue that what you see this early on isn't really a heartbeat at all, but a primitive or proto heartbeat, as the heart isn't fully formed yet and doesn't have its four pumping chambers. Instead, what can be seen on an ultrasound scan at this stage is a flickering electrical pulse as the hollow tube of cells that will eventually become the heart contracts. This 'beating' isn't actually audible at this stage, either. It's generally accepted that this cardiac activity happens for the first time around twenty-two to twenty-three days after conception – the beginning of the fifth week of pregnancy – which means, technically, this heartbeat may be there a few days before a scan can pick it up. Most clinics will only perform an ultrasound from six weeks, and even then the absence of a visible heart flicker is not always considered conclusive proof of a miscarriage. Often, they'll send you away for a week or so before repeating the scan.

Just because we can't see something doesn't mean it's not there. And yet, we tend to outsource our understanding of what is and isn't a pregnancy – *alive* – to technological proof and what we can visualize on a screen. But there are lots of reasons a heartbeat (or something akin to a heartbeat) could be present and still evade our probing. Someone's weight, the existence of scar tissue in the womb, how full the bladder is, or the position of the embryo can all affect how easily an early heartbeat can be detected. And a scan is only as good as the person performing it. Ditto the calibre and age of the scanning machine itself. In the 1980s, for example, when ultrasound first became a routine part of maternity care, women were advised that a heartbeat was only reliably visible from about eight weeks of pregnancy.

Being able to see a heartbeat on an ultrasound scan is, then, a relatively arbitrary marker. It's potentially consistent neither with the heart's first activity nor its completed development.

While the heart *is* the first organ to develop during pregnancy, and its characteristic four chambers take shape astonishingly early, at eight weeks, pioneering research that looked at scans of living foetal hearts has found that the heart muscle isn't fully developed, and doesn't function in an organized way, until twenty weeks – halfway through a typical pregnancy. This was much later than the team of scientists from the University of Leeds had anticipated and appears to set us apart, in terms of the timeline of our development, from other mammals.[1]

Which is all to say that, although this proof of a heartbeat feels infinitely significant to people like me and Dan, it isn't really any sort of threshold at all. It perhaps says more about our technological capability than anything fundamental about what makes us human.* It feels like an unsolvable riddle: can there be a heartbeat if there isn't yet a heart? What did your heart sound like before it was made? Personally, I find it hard to think of what we hope to see on the scan as anything other than a heartbeat. Today, if there is any evidence of that electrical activity – the flow of calcium ions in and out of heart cells, which a scan picks up as a coordinated flutter – it means that our dream of parenthood is alive. For now.

Although I know that our NHS clinic for recurrent-miscarriage patients will scan me at six weeks, I've waited a whole week longer this time. I'm not sure why. Perhaps because we've seen six-week-old heartbeats in three out of four

---

* Not that any of this has stopped anti-choice, 'right to life' proponents in several states in America trying to use it as the basis for restrictive anti-abortion legislation, the point at which it becomes illegal to terminate a pregnancy – sometimes including in instances of rape, incest, or serious foetal anomalies. Even before the overturning of Roe *v.* Wade in 2022, in Texas this 6-week limit was, functionally, the law. Although such laws have been nicknamed 'heartbeat bills', such is the medical nuance surrounding hearts and heartbeats, the American College of Obstetricians and Gynaecologists argues that we shouldn't call them this 'because it is misleading language, out of step with the anatomical and clinical realities of that stage of pregnancy'.

previous pregnancies, only for them to stop a few weeks later. Perhaps delaying by a week feels like breaking a pattern. Lucky number seven?

We step out of the Tube on to the dismal thoroughfare, in an area of the city that is neither cool nor sexy, not grand, and not plate-glass-shiny either. A pigeon-grey corridor that always seems to be under construction; all roadworks, bored faces, and chain restaurants.

We are early, so the first task is to find somewhere to get breakfast that we haven't been to before. Not the bland cafe-cum-sandwich bar that once served us thin, grey coffee before the thin, grey disappointment of inconclusive test results. And not the photogenic canal-boat restaurant where we ate Instagram-perfect, maple-syrup-soaked French toast half an hour before our fourth miscarriage was confirmed. We head down a side street and, as we walk, someone's second-hand cigarette smoke catches me at the back of the throat, as it always does when I'm pregnant. It's as hot and pungent as if I were smoking it myself, but I try to ignore it. I will not take this as a sign. I will not romanticize. This is not proof of a person already asserting their likes and dislikes. That's not how this works.

We end up at a cafe that seems to be attached to a boutique hotel, full of confident men with neat beards holding breakfast meetings. I order plain toast and overcooked bacon and a glass of orange juice. The thought of my usual cappuccino – decaf, naturally – turns my stomach. *That's new*, I think, before forcing my mind shut, like a trap. I will not convince myself that I feel 'more' pregnant than the other times. I know, rationally, that I've felt very pregnant before and it has come to nothing. But it's strange how a diagnosis of a miscarriage can make you a revisionist. You start unravelling the very fact of your pregnancy, unmaking its history, discounting the evidence of it, as though it were somehow less real to begin with. What if there is no heartbeat today? Will I have been any less pregnant? Will it *feel* like less of a pregnancy? Will it feel like less of a miscarriage? Will the disappointment be any different? The answer, I think, is both yes and no.

There's still a huge amount we don't know about the very earliest stages of pregnancy. So much so, the phase in between conception and when it can be visualized on a scan is sometimes referred to as the 'black box' of human development. When you lose a pregnancy in this unseen space, the void inevitably fills with doubt and anxiety over the ambiguous nature of your pregnancy and what happened to it. It clouds your judgement of what you are 'allowed' to feel. All miscarriages can trigger what Dr Kenneth Doka first described as 'disenfranchised grief'. That is, they are often 'losses that cannot be openly acknowledged, socially validated, or publicly mourned'.[2] As the eminent bereavement specialists Colin Murray Parkes and Holly G. Prigerson have noted, despite the distress it can cause, 'the death of a foetus rarely causes people to seek psychiatric help'.[3] And what if there never was a visible foetus? What if a scan shows only a pregnancy sac, without an embryo? What if the pregnancy isn't implanted in the womb at all, but out of place (ectopic)? What if you have a positive pregnancy test, but your period arrives shortly after, any embryo vanishing sight-unseen? In these circumstances, your loss is disenfranchised all over again. You find yourself in the peculiar position of wondering if you are grieving something that never really was.

Professor Nick Macklon is the medical director of the London Women's Clinic and a leading international authority on early pregnancy. He is one of the authors of a key piece of research – now twenty years old – titled 'Conception to ongoing pregnancy: the "black box" of early pregnancy loss'.[4] His work has been instrumental in crowbarring open this box, just a tiny bit, shedding light on this stage of pregnancy, what happens, and, in turn, what it means for infertility treatment and miscarriage. 'What that title alluded to was the difficulty we have in understanding what the fate is of the fertilized egg "in vivo", that is, in a normal situation, inside the body,' he explains. 'Pregnancy is an iceberg,' he continues. 'We only see the live births and the clinical miscarriages above the sea water, but there's much more underneath there.'

At the heart of this redacted section in our biology seems to be a quirk that's unique to humans. Unlike other animals, we have a very high attrition rate when it comes to pregnancy. Contrary to what we tend to believe about where babies come from, it is not actually as simple as sperm plus egg equals a baby in nine months' time. 'The proportion of fertilized eggs that turn into babies is very low,' Professor Macklon tells me. In fact, as his research concluded, as many as 60 per cent of all fertilized eggs (that is, very early-stage pregnancies or embryos) are rejected by the body before the period arrives – around half of those are lost before they implant in the womb and half after.[5] A further 10 per cent of all conceptions are then thought to be lost as clinically recognized miscarriages, or later losses, which means that out of all the sperm-meets-egg moments, just 30 per cent result in a live birth.

Why should this be? Why are the majority of conceptions lost at such an early stage? It's believed to be down to our comparatively high rate of chromosomal errors. As many as 20 per cent of egg cells and 9 per cent of sperm are thought to be abnormal in this way, even in healthy people.[6] 'This is different from other species,' says Professor Macklon. (In mice, for example, it's more like one in 200 cells that have these errors. In *Drosophila*, or fruit flies, it's one in 6,000.[7]) 'There's a discussion to be had about why we evolved in that way,' he adds. One theory is that there are benefits for humans to spacing out pregnancies over time that justify having this high rate of loss, rather than having a baby every nine months – as would potentially happen if practically every fertilized egg resulted in an ongoing pregnancy, indiscriminately. After all, unlike other

species, human babies are slow to wean and slow to reach physical maturity; they are, in other words, an expensive biological
undertaking. It makes sense that our bodies would have a high
threshold for the future children they choose to invest in. Yet
the idea of the female body as an active player in its reproductive fate, picking and choosing which embryos to take in, goes
against centuries of conditioning that tells women they are the
passive sex: done to, never doing.

These pre-clinical, pre-period losses are sometimes referred to
as 'occult' pregnancies. In medicine, 'occult' simply means symptomless, or unseen, though the term in this context does little to
counter the sense that this earliest phase of pregnancy is somehow less real and not of this world. A more familiar term to those
trying to conceive is a 'chemical pregnancy', or sometimes 'biochemical pregnancy', usually used to indicate that someone has
had a positive pregnancy test, meaning they have sufficiently
raised levels of the pregnancy hormone HCG but their period
arrives a week or even two weeks after – before a scan could
detect any sign of the pregnancy. 'Essentially it means there are
chemical signs of pregnancy, but no other ones,' explains Professor Macklon. But where does an 'occult' pregnancy end and a
'chemical pregnancy' begin? For that matter, at what point does
a chemical pregnancy become a miscarriage? Sometimes, women
talking about their experiences in furtive corners of the internet
differentiate between 'just a chemical' and a 'proper' miscarriage.
But is there a clear boundary between the two?

'Not really,' says Professor Macklon, who believes the term
'chemical pregnancy' is not a useful one. 'It's not very helpful for
patients,' he tells me. Not least because there is some debate
among scientists and professional organizations as to its strict
definition. 'There's a shared agreement on the concept, but around
the edges of terminology there's a lot of discussion,' he says.
'Some might say a biochemical pregnancy is not one that's got far

enough for us to consider it a miscarriage. My view is that any pregnancy that has been recognized by a woman has been present and then, if it doesn't continue, it's a clinical miscarriage.'

These earliest kinds of pregnancy losses have been labelled a 'new reproductive experience'[8] by anthropologists, one that has effectively been manufactured by the highly sensitive pregnancy tests that are available today, which work days *before* someone's period is due. Even just a few decades ago, the most sensitive tests could only confirm a pregnancy around nine days *after*. But while it may be true that technology has created these early experiences of loss, it does not mean we should dismiss them. These kinds of pregnancy losses may not have existed for our grandmothers' generation – or even our mothers' – but we cannot put the genie back in the bottle; we cannot un-know what it is now possible to know. 'It's an early pregnancy loss in my view and is going to be experienced as a disappointment,' agrees Professor Macklon. He sees it as part of a 'continuum' – one that starts with unsuccessful IVF transfers, a scenario in which someone knows a conception has taken place, that a fertilized egg has been placed back into their uterus, and will then know if it doesn't continue as a pregnancy. By comparison, a couple trying to conceive naturally will be unaware of this, even though on many occasions when a woman's period arrives on time, a fertilized egg may well have been lost.

What we don't yet know is whether these earliest forms of miscarriage are closer in nature to the pre-clinical, pre-period conception losses – in that they are, perhaps, a built-in part of our human biology, a fundamentally healthy sign – or whether they are losses that indicate something is going awry, especially if they happen repeatedly. Women are, unfortunately, still sometimes told that these earliest losses 'do not count' when it comes to being referred for further investigations for multiple miscarriages. Or they are told 'not to test so early' next time.

As Dan and I sit in the waiting room at the recurrent-miscarriage clinic, I am well aware that all those positive pregnancy tests could still translate to nothing on screen. All morning, I've been trying to identify something about the way I feel. Now, as I wait, hands knotted in my lap, legs crossed, one foot tapping an erratic beat in mid-air, it hits me. It isn't only nerves and fear and desperate hope. There is something else curdling the mix. The possibility of there being no visible pregnancy today doesn't only feel like it would be sad, it feels like it could be humiliating – as if I have only imagined myself pregnant. And women have a long history of being made to feel shame for things that are 'all in their heads'.

Of course, that is not what an empty ultrasound today would actually mean. In fact, whatever has or has not happened, the activity inside my uterus in the weeks since I took that first positive pregnancy test has been momentous, potentially definitive: a period of embryonic development known as gastrulation. 'It is not birth, marriage or death, but gastrulation that is truly the most important time in your life,' or so declared the embryologist Lewis Wolpert.[9] Gastrulation begins around sixteen days after conception, a week or so after the fertilized egg implants in the lining of the womb. In this phase, the cells – which have multiplied rapidly from one egg cell and one sperm cell – begin to rearrange themselves from a single, uniform layer into several distinct layers of different types of cell, from which the different organs of the body can then form. This includes the placenta. In this key stage, 'there's a huge amount of dialogue going on between the embryo and the uterus', says Professor Macklon. Yet currently scientists are unable to 'listen in' on this crucial conversation.

Currently there is no way to study this phase in humans. It is not possible to study it during an ongoing pregnancy without harming the embryo; it can't be visualized on scans; nor is it possible to study through embryos grown in a lab, as scientists are not allowed to do this beyond fourteen days – just before gastrulation begins.* This fourteen-day limit quickly became the international standard after the first successful IVF treatment, in 1978, but for a long time fourteen days was a hypothetical boundary as scientists didn't know how to keep embryos alive artificially for this long anyway (for context, this is around nine days after the age at which embryos are put back into the womb in IVF treatment). But in 2016, two different research teams managed to sustain embryos for thirteen days for the first time, prompting scientists to make the case for the rules to change.

Since then, there have been repeated calls from scientists for the limit to be extended. A recurring strand of these arguments is that a relaxing of the regulations could help explain and potentially prevent miscarriages. Thanks to an exceptionally rare tissue donation, in 2021 scientists were, for the very first time, able to study how exactly an embryo's cells behave during gastrulation. A team from the University of Oxford and the Helmholtz Zentrum München, Germany, mapped out the gene expression (essentially the coded instructions a cell uses to do its job) of all 1,195 individual cells of an embryo that was believed to be between sixteen and nineteen days post-fertilization. The study was described as the 'Rosetta Stone' for developmental biologists, in terms of its potential to translate the unknown language of the embryo, acting as a foundational text for future research.[10] For now, though, this kind of research is unlikely to be repeated, as the fourteen-day rule is enshrined in law in the UK, as well as in many other countries, including

* The little we do know about this stage of pregnancy in humans is based on either research on animals or historical specimens from human studies that would no longer pass modern ethical standards for research. For example, the last time doctors got to see gastrulation in action in humans was in experiments performed by gynaecologists in the 1950s and '60s who asked women due to have scheduled hysterectomies to have unprotected sex beforehand so the doctors could then study any early pregnancies found in the wombs that were removed.

Canada and Australia.* 'If we could accept as a society that we could keep embryos up to, say, twenty-two days, and it was technically possible, I think we would get some very useful information,' Professor Macklon tells me, 'because we could understand not just about the first five or six days, which we've learned a lot about, but what's really happening in those ten to twelve days after implantation starts – and this is key.' As well as understanding the pathway to miscarriage, such research could help improve IVF success rates, which, despite improving steadily over the years, still hover at just under a third of embryo transfers resulting in a baby. Half of embryos that implant in IVF do not make it to ongoing pregnancy, and yet 'the implantation process is a big black box for us clinicians', as Norbert Gleicher, head of the Center for Human Reproduction in New York, told the journal *Nature* in 2016.[11] If we could further unravel the mysteries of this stage of pregnancy – what goes wrong, and why – we could start to replace women's doubts, shame, and self-criticism with facts. *It was there. It was real. This is what happened to it.*

Sometimes, though, efforts to delineate the biology of earliest pregnancy, far from validating someone's feelings, can do the opposite – especially if the science is translated clumsily. Take, for example, an 'anembryonic' pregnancy, which is sometimes tactlessly referred to as a 'blighted ovum' (ovum meaning egg cell). This is diagnosed when the fluid-filled bag that an embryo develops inside – the gestational sac – can be seen on a scan but without any evidence of the embryo inside it. This absence of an embryo, of a *body*, can be particularly tormenting, as if it makes it a different, lesser category of miscarriage. 'I felt embarrassed

---

* Donated embryos at this stage of development are vanishingly rare, as many women do not know or realize they are pregnant this early on, especially if they are not actively trying to conceive. And donated embryos for research like this have to come from natural conceptions, which means scientists are reliant on tissue donated after pregnancies are terminated.

that I was so excited about the baby, sharing all my thoughts and stories with friends and family only to realise there was nothing there,' recounts one woman, writing on the Miscarriage Association's website. The spectre of this same embarrassment hovers over me now, still waiting to be called in for the scan.

Yet the idea that an anembryonic pregnancy is 'nothing' is an oversimplification. While it can leave us questioning whether what has happened was even a 'proper' miscarriage, it's been suggested that as many as 50 per cent of miscarriages are, in fact, anembryonic. It may even be the 'single leading cause' of miscarriage[12] (although it is hard to measure this precisely: if a miscarriage happens before a scan can take place, it may not be obvious either way whether an embryo was present). What's more, while the old-fashioned term 'blighted ovum' implies a fundamental flaw with the egg cell, one that meant no pregnancy started to develop, as the gynaecologist Professor Lesley Regan writes, 'more recent research studies suggest the apparently empty pregnancy sacs did contain an embryo at one time, but that the embryo was reabsorbed very early in its development'.[13] In other words, the idea that this kind of miscarriage is a failure to launch – a failing rooted in the woman's body thanks to a 'rotten' egg – is not based in biological reality. It is misogyny, handed down through language, not physiology.

Professor Macklon concurs. 'What we often see is a yolk sac [a structure that develops to provide the embryo with nutrition before the placenta forms] but no embryo – but the yolk sac comes from the embryo, so part of the embryo *has* developed and the other hasn't,' he explains. Personally, he says, he avoids using either 'blighted ovum' or 'anembryonic pregnancy' as he feels both terms have a 'judgemental undertone'. Instead, he favours the simpler and arguably kinder description 'the embryo has stopped developing early on'.

Without a cleaner, clearer medical understanding of the earliest steps of pregnancy, and until we change the unhelpful, obfuscating language – '*chemical*', '*blighted*', '*occult*' – used to describe it, an impression will remain that these earliest losses are a form of phantom pregnancy,* rather than a physical reality. Many of us will continue to be haunted by ideas that it was all in our head: that a chemical pregnancy is little more than a false positive result (exceptionally rare with modern pregnancy tests, for the record); that an IVF implantation 'failure' isn't really a loss; that an anembryonic pregnancy was somehow a figment of the womb's imagination. But it's pointless trying to stratify grief according to physical size, week of gestation, or whether you ever saw a heartbeat. Not least because sometimes a pregnancy can stop developing in the earliest black-box weeks, but the miscarriage won't be diagnosed until later, when someone believes they are eight, ten, or even twelve weeks along. Besides, the depth of feeling you have for a pregnancy isn't always rational, logical, or linear. The moment you see a second pink line on a pregnancy test, the possibility of your future child can expand mind-blowingly fast from nothing, Big Bang-like in its speed and scope.

At the recurrent-miscarriage clinic, Dan and I are finally called into the scanning room, after a long wait that feels longer. They ask you to come with a full bladder, so I am tetchy and uncomfortable. The waiting room is little more than a corridor and as far as I can tell the ultrasound room here isn't reserved only for

---

* In fact, 'phantom pregnancy' is a distinct medical phenomenon in its own right. Also called pseudocyesis – from the Greek for 'false' and 'pregnancy' – it's a condition in which a non-pregnant woman believes herself to be pregnant and develops objective signs of pregnancy, according to the American Psychiatric Association's *Diagnostic and Statistical Manual of Mental Disorders*, Fifth Edition (DSM-5). While the pregnancy may exist only in her head, a woman's stomach can swell, and her periods can stop. It is very rare, although it has been suggested that it's more common in cultures when a woman's worth and status are dependent on her ability to produce a child (https://www.ncbi.nlm.nih.gov/pmc/articles/PMC3674939/).

fertility patients like us, even on clinic days. There are other couples, and also women on their own, of all ages. There are no visible bumps, but a lot of blank faces, which I read as fear. It occurs to me, not for the first time, that a missing heartbeat might not be the only kind of bad news delivered here today.

We go in. I'm expecting to be sent straight out again to empty my bladder so they can do an internal ultrasound scan, with a probe, given how early it is. But, to my slight surprise, the sonographer wants to try through my abdomen first. I lie down on the bed covered with scratchy, NHS standard-issue blue paper and hold my breath. The gel goes on ('A little cold, sorry'). And there it is. That all-important flicker of white, on grey, on black. Barely bigger than a comma. But it is a comma, not a full stop. We exhale, though we do not celebrate or linger on this moment. It is far from a guarantee, it is just a shimmer on a screen, but it is indisputably, demonstrably, the start of something.

3

'It's just nature's way'

(November 2019 – 7–8 weeks pregnant)

After the scan, we get to see a consultant. We head into one of
the clinic's bland, square rooms, where we've sat before and
listlessly discussed 'management options' for a miscarriage or
nodded along as we're told there isn't really anything we can do
differently, other than try, try, try again. Only this time, I am
not sure I can just go along with things. Inertia and just-wait-
and-see don't feel like viable options this time. The need to
correct the course of this fifth pregnancy, to do anything and
everything within my power to protect it, surges through me –
electricity in my veins. I can feel it crouching in my muscles
and sinews. This time, I have a game plan. I am going to go
against my usual instincts, informed by the many weary doctors I've interviewed as a health journalist. I have done what I
know makes doctors' hearts sink to their shoes, and googled.
I've come to the appointment armed with study details and
statistics. I am going to be a Difficult Patient. I am going to
start a conversation with 'So, I read this thing online . . .'

Yet, I am still not particularly hopeful. It will not be the first time I have asked about some speculative treatment or theory that might explain what's happening to us – in the past, I've pressed doctors about the possibility of prescribing blood-thinning medication, steroids, or whether my miscarriages could be a sign of early menopause, among other things. So far, though, my suggestions and desperate hypotheses about why I can't hold on to a pregnancy have been kindly, but firmly, dismissed.

That our doctors have not prescribed so much as a single pill, after four miscarriages, is something that continues to surprise people who know us. 'What about IVF ... would that help?' friends and family have asked, their faces crumpling in confusion. No, I have had to explain, sometimes gently, sometimes less so, struggling to bite back my frustration. No, I am not infertile – not technically, anyway. *Getting* pregnant is not the issue. It is the *staying*-pregnant part that my body does not seem able to do. IVF, which attempts to solve fertility problems by ensuring sperm meets egg, will not encourage an embryo to stick around. And as far as our doctors – specialists, no less – are concerned, there is nothing else to be done. There is, as far as they can tell, nothing 'wrong' with me; no reason why I couldn't carry a baby to term without medical intervention. It is, however, almost impossible to truly believe this, given our track record.

This, then, is the first major impasse when it comes to medicine and miscarriage. There is a fundamental quandary when it comes to treating it – which is, whether we should treat it at all.

When you have a miscarriage, you learn two things in quick and quietly devastating succession. One: this happens all the time. 'It's really, really common,' a midwife or sonographer will tell you. Two: no one is going to try to find out why it happened. 'It's just one of those things,' they will say, as they pat your hand and pass the tissues, before sending you on your way. The impression that forms as you leave – perhaps with a hospital-strength sanitary pad wadded between your legs, perhaps clutching a leaflet for a support charity – is how little anyone seems to care about what has happened and why. You are made to feel that a miscarriage is so commonplace and so unavoidable that it isn't worth worrying about, talking about for long, or indulging with much medical brainpower. Currently, in the UK, it is only considered worth investigating possible causes after you have had three losses in a row.

Which is why, after my first miscarriage, what I felt, along-side the shock, disappointment, and cavernous emptiness, was cheated. Cheated, because when you're pregnant you are bombarded with instructions that are supposed to prevent this very thing. No unpasteurized cheese. No rare meat. No drinking. Don't smoke or dye your hair, and limit your caffeine intake – actually, better not to have any at all, if you can possibly help it. No cleaning out the cat's litter tray. Wear gloves if you're gardening. On and on it goes, a gauntlet of good behaviour. *Good, better, best.* I had, on some level, assumed that this meant we knew how to prevent miscarriage these days, that we understood why it happened and what caused it; that it could be all but avoided if you followed the rules.

But in those raw moments after you're told that there is no heartbeat, or that your womb is, once again, empty, you're slammed with the realization that the truth is more complicated than you knew. After a miscarriage, no one asks about what you ate, or whether you might have accidentally had a full-caff cappuccino or two. Instead, you find that miscarriage is largely judged to be beyond our control. More than that, it's accepted as part of the natural order of things, an unfortunate part of the cycle of healthy reproduction. The prevailing assumption is that 'it's just nature's way'. You are told – repeatedly – that 'it's just bad luck'. *Just one of those things. Just try again.*

Just, just, just.

The full implications of this unfolded slowly in the weeks

after my first miscarriage. The reality that I was not going to be told why this had happened, or whether it was likely to happen again, confronted me every time I went to change yet another sanitary pad, as my womb continued to shrink and shed long after that morning in A&E. The bleeding went on for so long, days leaking into weeks, that when I no longer needed to go out with a pad in, I felt a hiccup of something akin to happiness for the first time since; it almost felt like a milestone. At last it was *really* over.

Before I was pregnant, or even wanted to be, the idea that miscarriage was essentially natural and therefore couldn't be prevented would have struck me as intuitively correct, if I'd stopped to consider it at all. The belief that miscarriage is nature's form of quality control, which saves us from further heartache and loss of life later on – cruel, but ultimately kind – is one that runs deep. And there is, of course, some truth in it. For many women, a miscarriage will be a one-off event, a result of a random, unsurvivable chromosomal error. For some, there may even be a modicum of comfort in thinking along these lines. Yet, to assume that a miscarriage is always 'for the best' and therefore without consequence is wrong. Quite apart from the emotional impact of having the expected course of your life so brutally turned about, there may be other, longer-term health consequences, such as an increased risk of pre-term birth in subsequent pregnancies, which rises incrementally with every miscarriage a person has.[1]

The assumption that miscarriage is normal and inevitable – preferable, even, if the alternative is a desperately, incurably ill baby – feels very different from the other side of the looking glass. The day after that first loss, my mum came to see us.

'You don't have to do anything. We don't have to go anywhere. But I want to come and sit with you,' she'd insisted, over text.

We ended up in John Lewis. Ostensibly, we went because I

needed a new winter coat, my old one having been stained beyond the skill of any dry cleaner – as much to do with memory as with blood. Really, I think we went because I knew the department store would feel safe, predictable, clean, and quiet, in a way that the day before hadn't been. John Lewis: nothing very bad could happen to you there. In the changing-room mirrors, my face was pale and bloodless; my stomach somehow deflated and too large at the same time. After an hour or so of browsing, we went for coffee: my first proper caffeine in months. Later, when Mum took me and Dan out for dinner, I had a glass of wine. The first sip made me want to cry, dissolved by the knowledge that I was 'allowed' to drink again. *Too soon.* I wanted to scream at the people at the next table, in our local Italian: 'I shouldn't be doing this – I should still be pregnant!'

Mum convinced me to ask for time off work. I emailed my editor, opting for honesty, all the while unsure whether it really was the best policy. There was no page in the employee handbook on miscarriage. What did I need? What was allowed? Was one day off enough? Was three excessive? Fortunately, my boss urged me to take the whole week. I didn't get dressed. I lay down a lot, but didn't sleep easily. I don't remember what I ate or drank. I wanted to disappear. Or better yet, go back in time. A few days in, I watched an old episode of *Sex and the City*, in which Charlotte has a miscarriage, which had been plaguing me like an earworm. I paused and rewound, analysing every line, incredulous that the matter was dispatched in so few minutes of screen time, irrationally furious that this was my main reference point for a miscarriage and that it had prepared me so poorly for my own. When I wasn't on the sofa, I sat at my computer writing and writing: streams of bitter, heartbroken words going nowhere. Towards the end of the week, I took myself to the canal for a run. Thanks to first-trimester tiredness, I had not done this for months. My body felt heavy, waterlogged, and after a mile or so my knee ached – an old injury playing up, but also, I knew, a possible effect of lingering pregnancy hormones.* The baby may have been gone, but my ligaments and joints hadn't got the memo. I forced myself to keep going. I was not pregnant any more, so fuck the antenatal health warnings about susceptibility to injury. *Fuck biology*, I thought. I ran hard, harder than felt safe or sensible, conscious of the softness of my stomach with every step, each reverberation of extra flesh a taunt. *Fuck Mother Nature.*

There are many other events and ailments in life that could be considered 'nature's way' and yet, unlike miscarriage, we do not accept them with the shrugging indifference of 'just, just, just'. Failing joints, age-related hearing loss, even crooked teeth. We do not accept dementia as an inevitable and therefore acceptable price of an ageing population. We replace worn-out hips and dispel the fog of cataracts. We vaccinate against pneumonia – an illness that was not so long ago nicknamed the 'old man's friend'. An extraordinary amount of money and research-time has been spent ensuring men can have erections long after nature might consider that an expendable pleasure.†
In almost every other area of medicine, nature is considered far

---

* The levels of a hormone called relaxin rise each month after ovulation, increasing if a pregnancy is conceived. It's produced by the ovaries and then the placenta once that forms. Most women are told about its role in preparing the pelvis for birth – essentially it loosens everything up so something large can fit through somewhere that is normally quite narrow – but it can have a knock-on effect on other muscles and joints around the body. Interestingly, though, relaxin's function is more complicated than this. Levels are highest in the first trimester, and some researchers have suggested it is likely 'an important player in early pregnancy maintenance' with both too much and too little being a potential problem. More recently, it's been suggested by scientists in the Netherlands that there may be a link between low levels of circulating relaxin in the first trimester and the condition pre-eclampsia in later pregnancy.
† Before it became available over the counter in 2018, there were almost 3 million prescriptions for erectile dysfunction each year in the UK. Just saying.

too cruel a mistress to preside in an advanced society. But quite apart from the fact that we do not apply the same Darwinian standards to other areas of health, the idea that miscarriage is almost always down to a fundamental, unpreventable error written into the building blocks of our human code is not the full story. 'Not all miscarriages are the same,' explains Arri Coomarasamy, a professor of gynaecology and reproductive medicine, and the director of the UK's National Centre for Miscarriage Research, set up by the charity Tommy's in 2016. 'There is this myth out there that every miscarriage that occurs is because of some profound problem with the pregnancy, that there's nothing that can be done.' But science, he says, is finally starting to 'unpick that myth'.

In the same editorial that called for 'worldwide reform' of miscarriage care, published in the *Lancet* medical journal in 2021, it was suggested that an assumption that miscarriage is natural and warrants little to no medical intervention is 'ideological, not evidence based'. The editorial introduced a series of research papers in that issue that attempted to outline the scale of the problem, the known risk factors for miscarriage, and possible treatments, as well as the important – yet undervalued – repercussions of pregnancy loss. 'What we know is that roughly half of miscarriages take place because there is a serious problem with the foetus,' says Professor Coomarasamy, who is one of the authors of the *Lancet* series. 'But we also know that the other half of pregnancies don't have such problems. Those are called euploid miscarriages and the other group, the ones with chromosomal problems, are called aneuploid miscarriages. Those euploid miscarriages, they can and should be prevented.' The language of 'nature's way' and 'just one of those things', he adds, 'misses the point – there are so many miscarriages that needn't take place, but they do'.

That as many as half of all miscarriages are of healthy, 'normal' pregnancies is not brand-new information. Patient-support leaflets since at least as far back as the 1980s have offered up this 50 per cent statistic as a possible explanation for why miscarriages happen.[2] Why is it only now that more doctors and researchers are highlighting that such a significant proportion of losses have the potential to be spared? Part of the problem, perhaps, has been the knowledge that a miscarriage is likely to be a one-off event, with the majority of people going on to have a successful pregnancy the next time they conceive.[3] Accordingly, the guiding philosophy has been that not only is miscarriage something that cannot be fixed – it doesn't *need* to be fixed. It's true that around 80 per cent of people who have one miscarriage will go on to have a baby at the next attempt – though, to look at it another way, this means that after one miscarriage, the chance of another does rise to 20 per cent, from 5 per cent if you have never been pregnant or had a miscarriage before. A miscarriage is not a statistically meaningless event.[*]

Yet, in the aftermath of a single miscarriage, the line between what is 'normal' and what is considered a medical problem is presented to you as a stark boundary. One is nothing to worry about, two is also probably fine. It's only when you get to three that it might become something requiring action, in as much as tests should be offered to check for certain known issues, something which generally requires a referral to a specialist clinic. In reality, the distinction is much more porous. Even when it comes to recurrent miscarriage – that is, those who have three or more miscarriages in a row – doctors will not suddenly go in

---

[*] It took a surprisingly long time for doctors to establish this. It was the mid-1980s before Professor Lesley Regan designed a study – the Cambridge Miscarriage Study – to look at this issue, after finding that the available evidence at the time unhelpfully put the risk of another miscarriage at anything between 15 per cent and 75 per cent. The results of this study, which also showed that having a previous termination did not increase the risk of a subsequent miscarriage, were published in 1989 (see note 3).

all guns blazing. You may well be told that your prospects are still very good, that for just over half of people who've lost three pregnancies in a row, the next one will stick – even without treatment. This, though, is one of those trickster statistics – capable of appearing to be perfectly good odds to a dispassionate clinician, while simultaneously looking decidedly like a losing hand when you're the one sitting in the other chair, trying to have the baby. A near 50 per cent chance of having yet another miscarriage is hard to swallow as a reason to be optimistic, and to justify not taking further medical action.

The reasoning behind waiting for miscarriage to become 'recurrent' before offering investigations and – possibly – treatment, is that when this happens it's more likely that the losses are down to something other than random, out-of-the-blue chromosomal disorders. But this doesn't track perfectly with the evidence, either. As Professor Coomarasamy tells me, 'For recurrent miscarriage, broadly speaking it's the same: roughly half are down to chromosomal problems.' To say that this complicates the picture is something of an understatement. To me, it seems to fly in the face of the foundational logic of who gets miscarriage follow-up care and who doesn't, undermining the notion that a single miscarriage is more likely to be down to a random coding error than to something that has the capacity to be prevented or treated. 'Even if someone has a sporadic [one-off] miscarriage, I don't think it's right to say it was probably chromosomal problems that caused it,' confirms Professor Coomarasamy.*

* There is, though, a caveat here, given the research available – or rather, the lack of it (a recurring theme in this area of medicine). 'The research is somewhat limited, in that we don't get to analyse all the pregnancy tissue of people who've had sporadic miscarriages,' explains Professor Coomarasamy, adding that data from older studies that has managed to look at genetic material from lost pregnancies will be based on older, now-outdated technology, which might make the results less accurate.

There is also disagreement within the medical community around the world as to what should count as recurrent loss, i.e. a clinical condition worthy of medical investigation as opposed to a natural and inevitable part of life. For some organizations, such as the European Society of Human Reproduction and Embryology (ESHRE) and the American Society for Reproductive Medicine, the definition has been revised down from three losses to two in recent years. However, for others, including the NHS, the UK's Royal College of Obstetricians and Gynaecologists, the Health Service Executive in Ireland, and the French College of Gynaecologists and Obstetricians, it remains three or more.* There were calls in spring 2021 from the authors of the *Lancet* research series, and from the charity Tommy's, which funded much of the work, for treatment for miscarriage to kick in at an earlier stage, with a more nuanced, graduated approach than currently exists in the UK. They recommended a 'graded model of care', which would involve an assessment after one miscarriage, and the offer of information and support for future pregnancies. After two, women would ideally be seen at a miscarriage clinic for blood tests and have early scans in subsequent pregnancies. After three, additional tests should be offered, such as genetic testing and pelvic ultrasound. However, as yet, the UK government has not taken up these recommendations.

'Miscarriage is horrible whether you have one, two, or three,' says Professor Nick Macklon, of the London Women's Clinic. 'We need to take it seriously and we need to understand miscarriage to be able to prevent it as much as possible.' However, he also issues a note of caution lest we 'generate false hope

---

* There are also variations in whether the losses have to be consecutive to warrant investigation, or whether multiple miscarriages are a cause for concern if they fall either side of healthy pregnancies, and whether particular types of loss, such as ectopic or molar pregnancy, should be included. Some suggest investigations should be done sooner if someone is over the age of thirty-five.

and expectation'. 'I'm not sure that medicalizing all miscarriage is going to be helpful,' he tells me, picking his words carefully, adding that the conversation needs to be more nuanced than a message that anyone who has one miscarriage has a medical problem that the NHS needs to diagnose and treat. 'I don't believe that's the case,' he says. 'Some women will go on to have recurrent miscarriages. Is there any way we can identify them early on? I think there is something in that.' However, ultimately, he believes some early miscarriages really are, regrettably, 'nature's quality control'. 'The obvious consequence of making embryos stick when they shouldn't is that you cause catastrophe further down the line,' he says. 'We have the same issue when we talk about recurrent implantation failure in IVF. We're all trying to make every embryo implant, because that will make our patients happy, but are we just converting implantation failure into miscarriage?' In other words, the uncomfortable truth is probably that some miscarriages can be prevented, while others can't – or shouldn't be. 'But we need to make that differentiation,' concludes Professor Macklon.

As it stands, though, we treat everyone who has one miscarriage the same way – in that we don't treat them at all. We have no way of ascertaining who will go on to have multiple miscarriages and whose is likely to have been a one-off. We don't even attempt to determine which 'type' of miscarriage it was – whether there was a chromosomal problem or not. For consultant obstetrician Professor Siobhan Quenby, who is also an author of the *Lancet* research series, finding out whether you are losing chromosomally 'normal' or abnormal pregnancies should be a key question in miscarriage care. Because what might help someone who has lost, say, two healthy, 'euploid' embryos in a row and what might help someone who has lost three successive aneuploid pregnancies are potentially very different things. 'Everybody's obsessed with counting the number of miscarriages, but to me it's ridiculous just to count the number – we should be looking at whether it was a normal or abnormal embryo,' she tells me.

Research into miscarriage rarely distinguishes between these two 'types' of loss, either, which has the potential to muddy the waters of what we know. Professor Quenby, for one, is unconvinced that, for people who have recurrent loss, the pattern is always random, with a roughly equal chance of a miscarried embryo being chromosomally normal or not. 'I'm fairly certain that people either recurrently lose abnormal ones or they recurrently lose normal ones,' she says. 'But that's only my opinion at the moment – it's something we'll have to work on.' As a bare minimum, 'everyone from their third miscarriage onwards should have their miscarriage tissue tested genetically,' she adds, as this could be a clue to what is happening in their individual case. However, access to such genetic testing – sometimes referred to as karyotyping – is patchy. Not everyone is told such testing is available to them. Indeed, not all NHS hospitals can do this kind of testing on site. And if someone miscarries at home, the onus is on them to collect a clean sample of the tissue and take it to the right part of their local hospital within twenty-four hours. Again, this may not be something they are able to do – or are told is an option.

When it comes to the key question of how many miscarriages can be prevented and how many can't, we seem to be very far from knowing where the dividing line actually is. Both Professor Coomarasamy and Professor Quenby suggest to me that a key reason we don't know more about miscarriage is a fundamental lack of motivation, verging on nihilism. To me, to continue to be so fatalistic about it seems against the spirit of science. After all, history suggests we are not very good at judging what is and isn't biological inevitability. It wasn't until

several decades into the twentieth century that any attempt at all
was made to save the lives of premature babies. Before that, back
when simple medical problems like diarrhoea or skin infections
could be fatal, the deaths of thousands of babies and young children each year were similarly considered 'just nature's way'.
Even the most pioneering of doctors once believed a large number of such deaths were – and always would be – inevitable due
to the innate, unconquerable fragility of small humans. Admittedly, sometimes after a miscarriage what you want, more than
anything, is the impossible: for the pregnancy to be reinstated,
remade, returned to you. Still, how can we be so certain we've
reached the ceiling of our ability to preserve life? Because, when
it comes to preventing miscarriage, it feels to me we've barely
begun even to try.

If making sense of a miscarriage when it happens to you often
feels a swirling, confusing endeavour, like trying to catch smoke
with your fingers, it's partly because you are, knowingly or not,
running up against potentially huge questions: questions about
the limits of what medicine can and should set out to achieve;
questions about the nature of illness and pathology; questions
about what is essential human nature that we would be wise not
to interfere with. Here's what Dan and I know, as it stands, in
these earliest weeks of our fifth pregnancy. Three of our miscarriages are unexplained. One – the fourth – was down to a
confirmed chromosomal error. The testing required to find this
out was only offered to us because we qualified as recurrent-
miscarriage patients by then – and because we knew to ask for it.
Specifically, the pregnancy was found to have an issue known as
a triploidy. This is where the embryo has inherited an extra set
of chromosomes, meaning each cell has an additional set of
these genetic instructions, totalling 69 rather than the usual 46.
Triploidies are random errors, rather than down to anything in
either parent's genes, and they are thought to account for
approximately a fifth of all first-trimester miscarriages that stem

from chromosomal abnormalities. It is exceptionally rare for babies with triploidy to survive to the second trimester (after thirteen weeks of pregnancy), even rarer for them to survive until birth and, if they do, to live for more than a few hours. The extra set of chromosomes can come from the egg cell, the sperm cell, or – most commonly – because two normal sperm happened to fertilize the egg at the same time. Two sperm and an unfortunate split second in time: miscarriage really can be as random and uncontrollable as that.

I learned that this had been the fate of our fourth pregnancy over the phone, several weeks after the miscarriage had been confirmed the previous year. I'd been at work. As I listened to the unfamiliar doctor tasked with explaining the results to me, I paced the back corridor by the lifts, like everyone did when they got a personal phone call, trying their best to pretend that life – with all its inconvenient diagnoses, heartbreaks, and burst pipes – didn't exist beyond the office walls. As I hung up, I felt short-lived relief. It was a definitive explanation, at least. Then I realized the information was going to make no difference at all to 'next time'. Given the random nature of this fourth loss, and with no other medical leads, the working theory was that our miscarriages really had been 'just bad luck'. A string of different, unrelated chromosomal errors, perhaps. With that fourth attempt, at least, had one sperm cell been just a fraction slower off the mark, our life could have been very different by now, possibly. Sex on a different night, or in a different position, could have meant we'd had a baby after all, maybe. Tens of millions of sperm cells can enter the uterus when a man ejaculates. Trying to understand the magnitude of these infinitesimal differences is dizzying, if you think about it for too long. It's like trying to grasp just how many stars there are in the galaxy – or how far away those thousands of billions of stars are from Earth.

Whichever way we look at things, though, Dan and I really do not have very much information to go on. But after our first miscarriage, we knew even less. All I was really certain of back then was my desperate, clawing desire to be pregnant again. I got my wish – and quickly, conceiving just three menstrual cycles later. I worked just that little bit harder at being pregnant this time. Whereas before, I'd carried on doing my usual exercise classes, albeit more gently and with a careful eye on a heart-rate monitor, this time nothing above walking pace felt safe. I drank no coffee at all, not even decaf. Still, underneath the caution was a confidence that this time it would work out. After all, hadn't we been told over and over that it was almost certainly a one-off? Even when we went for an early 'reassurance' scan, arranged by our sympathetic GP, and were told that the gestational sac was measuring a little small for seven weeks, I still hoped for the best, in a way I would find impossible now. The sonographer refused to be drawn on what the sac measurement might mean; perhaps they didn't know. The word miscarriage wasn't ever used. But we were told to come back in two weeks for a follow-up scan to see if it had 'caught up'. I almost pity that version of myself now, who didn't realize that the writing was almost certainly on the wall.*

The bleeding started a few days before the planned follow-up appointment. Just speckles of pink at first and then some bigger spots as the morning waxed on. We had friends staying for the bank holiday weekend, who took themselves off for a walk in the bright May sunshine while we went to the early-pregnancy unit. 'Just in case,' we told them. 'It's probably nothing.' Did I really, truly, naively believe that? Or was I just putting a positive spin on it for their sake? We'd only just told them the night before that I was pregnant again.

---

* In 2020, a study funded by the University of Tennessee Health Science Center, published in the journal *Scientific Reports*, suggested that after five completed weeks of pregnancy, a small gestational sac and a large yolk sac 'reliably predicted pregnancy loss'.

We were seen in the same room as last time, with the same midwife. She tilted the screen away in the same, tactful way. She gave us the same, tiny shake of the head. She delivered the same, half-whispered line: 'There is no heartbeat.' Numbness set in like fog, as we were handed more leaflets – the same leaflets we still had in the basket by the phone at home from our first visit, tucked under a layer of takeaway menus. This time, unlike before, the miscarriage wasn't 'complete', so we went home to wait it out. We begged our friends to stay for dinner, somehow reluctant to have all of our plans unmade. We sat out in the garden and put on a good show. Dan fired up the barbecue, while I served up performatively large, colourful cocktails. I didn't want to sit by myself in sadness this time. I wanted to laugh and clink glasses and pretend, just for an afternoon, that I didn't mind, that it wasn't happening. It wasn't *supposed* to happen, after all.

It was only later, when I excused myself to go to bed early, the bleeding having begun in earnest, that reality crept in. I spread an old beach towel over the bed, then I curled myself around a hot water bottle, willing sleep to find me. I woke an hour or so later, to short, sharp cramps and an insistent pressure in my vagina. I peeled off my pants and pad, and there it was: the embryo. This time, unlike last time, it was obvious what it was. It was perfectly intact, coiled and semi-lucent in its sac, a biology textbook come to life – almost. There was a poppy seed I took for an eye and nubs of limbs, like a tadpole. It was the size of the yolk from a chicken's egg and it didn't really look like a baby. It could never have lived outside of me. I knew this. But I badly wanted to resuscitate it anyway; to restart that tiny heart and palpate that chest, little broader than a thumb tip. Instead, I sat in the gathering dark of my bedroom, holding it in my palm, wanting to keep it with me just a little longer.

After two miscarriages, your chance of having another one increases slightly again, from 20 per cent to 24 per cent. After three it jumps to 43 per cent. From there, the risk increases slightly with every subsequent loss. After four, as much as Dan and I have been told we are still more likely than not to have a baby, eventually it feels as though we are on a slippery slope to hopelessness. After three or more miscarriages, and where the cause is unknown, an estimated six out of ten women will go on to have a baby the next time they conceive. This is presented to you as good news: no need to run yourself ragged searching for answers and new things to try. But it's all a matter of perspective, isn't it? Some have to be the four in ten: a 40 per cent chance of having yet another miscarriage and not a baby. You wouldn't get on a flight if that were your chance of a safe landing. You probably wouldn't even eat in a restaurant if you knew that was the risk of getting food poisoning.

Desperate to improve our odds, now that I am pregnant again, there is one treatment I am keen to try: progesterone. Progesterone has long been the great hope of miscarriage research, with trials into its effectiveness dating back to at least the 1950s. This 'pro-gestation' hormone is produced in higher quantities during pregnancy by a woman's ovaries and, later on, by the placenta. There is now some, albeit not overwhelming, evidence that taking additional progesterone may help increase the chance of having a live birth after previous miscarriages.

In between my fourth loss and this fifth pregnancy, in May 2019, a large, multi-centre trial of progesterone given in early pregnancy found that for women with a history of recurrent miscarriage who had started bleeding during their next pregnancy, taking progesterone made a significant difference to the live-birth rate, compared with a placebo.[4] I'd read about it online. 'If women had three or more previous miscarriages, there was a 15 per cent uplift in the live-birth rate,' Professor Coomarasamy, who led the research, tells me.

Previous trials with progesterone have been mixed, contra-dictory, or have shown no benefit at all, which is why, as I prepare to press my consultant about what I can do differently this time, it is not yet a routine part of NHS treatment for recurrent mis-carriage.* But this most recent study, known as the PRISM (progesterone in spontaneous miscarriage) trial, was far larger and more precisely designed than previous attempts. In Professor Coomarasamy's view, it was 'the largest, highest-quality trial' that had ever been done. 'It's nothing like what we had before,' he says. 'The largest of the previous trials had, maybe, 200 patients, whereas the PRISM trial had more than 4,000.'

Admittedly, the benefit for women who've had multiple mis-carriages was a secondary finding to the study's initial aims, involving a much smaller subset of women. The trial originally looked at whether there was any benefit in giving progesterone to *all* women who started bleeding in early pregnancy (referred to clinically as a threatened miscarriage, even though the bleed-ing can sometimes be innocuous). In this broader group, the researchers found no benefit. But for the group of 301 women in the PRISM trial who'd had three or more miscarriages, 72 per cent of those who took progesterone went on to have a baby, compared with 57 per cent of women in the placebo group.

A 15 per cent uplift: *15 per cent*. That looks and feels like a lifeline to me, right now. At the very least, the prospect of trying something different, something with even a scrap of evidence behind it, feels like it could keep me afloat psycho-logically, even if it can't save this pregnancy. In the consultant's office, I am prepared to go into battle for it. I know the new evidence for progesterone doesn't fit our circumstances

---

* This would finally change in November 2021, with the official guidance recom-mending that progesterone should be prescribed for anyone who starts bleeding during pregnancy if they've had at least one previous miscarriage. It's been esti-mated that this could lead to 8,450 more live births each year.

perfectly. I am not bleeding in this pregnancy, for one thing. And while there is a suspicion that, for women with my history, bleeding or otherwise, progesterone could be of benefit, 'the evidence is not absolutely clear-cut', says Professor Coomarasamy. 'It seems that for women who've had four or more miscarriages, even if they are not currently bleeding, progesterone might be of benefit. But there's some statistical uncertainty around that.' In other words, researchers have found a small increase in the live-birth rate, but not enough to publish a convincing academic paper to show it makes a difference.

To my surprise, the kind female doctor sitting across from us at the clinic today agrees to prescribe it without so much as a raised eyebrow. I haven't even had to rattle off the PRISM facts and figures that I have saved on my phone and imprinted in my brain before she nods.

'Yes, I think you'd be a good candidate for that,' she says.

As Dan and I join the queue at the hospital pharmacy, I am holding on to something far bigger than the printed prescription in my hand. For the first time, in what feels like such a long time, we have something, after being told that there was nothing.

Less than a week later, at eight weeks pregnant, I start to bleed.

4

'It's probably nothing'

(December 2019 – 8–9 weeks pregnant)

When you're pregnant and bleeding, the internet is a black hole; a vacuum, devoid of solid answers, yet there is no resisting its gravitational pull. When those all-too-familiar brownish-pink streaks start to appear, as much as I crave reassurance, I also know full well what I'll find online. For every anonymous story on a Mumsnet thread from someone who bled through their entire pregnancy and now has a strapping, six-foot twenty-two-year-old, there are just as many for whom bleeding was the beginning of the end. Worse still are the pages and pages of unanswered questions and inconclusive conversations. The internet is littered with these zombie threads, started by women who are bleeding, spotting, or cramping, at six, seven, eight, nine weeks. 'Any positive stories?' they ask, again and again, searching for hope in the experience of strangers. The replies – positive and negative – inevitably come flooding back and the original poster updates the forum for a bit: bleeding stopped, bleeding worse, no cramps yet, back pain, vag pain, bright-red blood, dark-brown blood, fresh blood, old blood – and then, very often, the thread falls quiet, with one last message: 'Got my scan tomorrow.' Then nothing. Contact is severed, like an astronaut falling out of reach of Mission Control.

Once more, I sift through the forums and threads. I am stunned and also entirely unsurprised that we are back here again. I am resigned to a fifth miscarriage and yet still pathetically hopeful as I skim the search results – the distress calls of so many others before me. *Any positive stories? Hi Ladies, losing hope over here tonight. Hi Ladies, Hi Ladies, Hi Ladies . . .*

This time, I do at least manage to establish that a relatively common side effect of the progesterone pessaries I'm now taking several times a day is bleeding. I learn this from IVF patient forums, quickly working out that supplementary progesterone is a standard medication given as part of that process. Apparently, progesterone can irritate the cervix (the neck of the womb), causing anything from watery, pink-tinged discharge to brown spotting.

The trouble is, this progesterone bleeding – if that's what it actually is – looks identical to the start of two of my previous miscarriages (the other two having been symptomless and diagnosed on scans). And, at eight weeks along, I am now at the precise stage my previous three pregnancies ended. Plus, no one at the clinic mentioned that this could be a possible side effect of the progesterone. It is, all things considered, very hard to believe this is anything but another miscarriage.

I know I should phone the recurrent-miscarriage clinic, or call my GP and perhaps try to get referred for a scan at my nearest early-pregnancy unit. But we have an appointment at the clinic booked in for the following Wednesday anyway – a fortnight on from our last scan – and we can discuss our options then, if need be. Meanwhile, my GP doesn't actually know that I'm pregnant yet and I can see little point in getting an emergency appointment at our local hospital, to sit in the same room and be told by the same midwife the same things we've heard before. Either there won't be a heartbeat, or we'll be given the discomfiting diagnosis of a 'threatened miscarriage', as all bleeding in early pregnancy is referred to clinically if a miscarriage or a related complication, such as an ectopic pregnancy, cannot be confirmed.

Bleeding in early pregnancy is common, with estimates suggesting it affects between one in four and one in five people before twenty weeks. This is roughly the same proportion as the number of pregnancies that end in miscarriage; though – perhaps counter-intuitively – it is not necessarily the same one in four or one in five who bleed who go on to have losses. While bleeding in pregnancy is the single biggest predictive factor for miscarriage, it does not mean a miscarriage will inevitably follow. In fact, some estimates have suggested that for around half of cases of bleeding, the pregnancy will continue, apparently unperturbed. Yet the term 'threatened miscarriage' is the one doctors use. Given that there is often little certainty as to what future your bleeding indicates, to me it's a label that manages to feel both imprecise and alarmist.

Bleeding in pregnancy can happen for a number of reasons. Very early on – around the time someone's period is due – it can be innocuous 'implantation' bleeding, a normal by-product as the embryo burrows into the womb lining. Later on, in the second and third trimesters, bleeding can be a sign of an issue with the position or function of the placenta. In the first trimester, it is commonly attributed to something called a subchorionic haemorrhage or haematoma (essentially a bleed or blood clot in the membranes around the baby). This can be seen on an ultrasound scan. Bleeding can also happen because the cervix becomes irritated or inflamed – after sex, for example, or due to an infection. Pregnancy hormones can also cause a benign growth of cervical cells called ectropion, which can bleed. And, of course, bleeding can be the start of a miscarriage, as the womb starts to unmake what it had previously made.

Sometimes, though, medics are unable to provide specifics – whether through a lack of concrete knowledge, or a lack of capacity in a stretched system. Sometimes, bleeding in pregnancy can happen for no discernible reason, and the pregnancy will be fine; at others, the pregnancy will end, if not right away, then at some later point. In that last scenario, whether the earlier bleeding was significant, or unrelated, will remain unknown. As gynaecologist and miscarriage specialist Professor Lesley Regan eloquently writes, 'Miscarriage is a process, not a single event.'[1]

The trouble is, we don't fully understand all the steps and warning signs along the way. Meanwhile, the things that *are* known aren't always communicated very well. As vague and unsatisfying as the diagnosis of 'threatened miscarriage' feels when it's happening to you, medically speaking there are strict criteria as to when it can be offered. It's given when there is a confirmed, apparently ongoing pregnancy in the womb, there has been some bleeding and/or abdominal pain, but the neck or opening of the womb – the cervix – remains closed. The cervix remaining closed is key. 'If we scan or examine someone and find the neck of the womb is open, unfortunately it is highly likely that a miscarriage will occur,' explains Dr Christine Ekechi, a consultant obstetrician and gynaecologist at Queen Charlotte's and Chelsea Hospital in London, who is the lead for ultrasound training in early pregnancy at her hospital. This is sometimes then referred to as an 'inevitable' miscarriage.

When a miscarriage is only 'threatened' rather than 'inevitable', attempting to answer the all-important question of how likely it is that the threat will come good – or perhaps, more accurately, come *bad* – is less straightforward. For those who find themselves in this scenario, it can be 'a very traumatic and anxiety-provoking time', says Dr Ekechi. 'People, understandably, want us to give definitive answers. But we cannot give definitive answers. And that's one of the difficulties with early pregnancy: managing expectations.'

Accepting that in medicine as a whole there are 'very few absolutes', as Dr Ekechi puts it, in early pregnancy there are still 'significant limitations' as to what doctors know, and even more so when it comes to how they can intervene. 'Early pregnancy is a specialty that has not been given a lot of credence for many, many years,' says Dr Ekechi, 'although that is changing. Just because a woman has not reached twenty-four weeks does not make a pregnancy less valuable, and therefore the amount of effort and research that has previously been put into understanding obstetrics should now equally be put into understanding miscarriage and early pregnancy.'

In the UK today, an estimated 60 per cent of babies born extremely prematurely, at twenty-four weeks – the threshold of 'viability' – will survive.[2] Treatment is not always beyond the realms of possibility or hope even if a baby is born at just twenty-two or twenty-three weeks. Yet this is a relatively recent reality. Until the 1990s, the limit of viability – that is, the point at which doctors could and would intervene – was set a full month later than it is now, at twenty-eight weeks. If pregnancies ended before this point, they were considered late miscarriages, whereas now they would be counted and treated as stillbirths or neonatal deaths. But compared with the remarkable advancements that have been made in later pregnancy and neonatal medicine, Dr Ekechi warns, early pregnancy is 'much more complicated and nuanced', and so progress, even with more investment and research interest, is likely to be more tentative. 'In early pregnancy, we're talking about cells that are still rapidly dividing; the organs have not yet developed; it's very fragile. So, what we may or may not be able to achieve is going to be very different. I don't necessarily think it's impossible, I just think it's a harder hill to climb,' she adds.

In the future, it may be that we will have reliable biomarkers that enable doctors to determine whether bleeding is the onset

of miscarriage or not. For example, there is some evidence that
blood levels of the protein CA-125, more commonly known as
a tumour-marker for ovarian cancer, can accurately predict
whether someone's pregnancy will continue. In pregnancy,
CA-125 is produced by the decidua – the layer of the uterus lining that adapts in preparation to support a baby. If an embryo
starts to detach from the decidua, it seems that CA-125 is then shed
into the pregnant person's bloodstream. Therefore, if someone's levels are high, it may indicate miscarriage, while if their
levels are low, it's more likely a pregnancy will continue.[3]
However, more research is needed to confirm and finesse such
a test for mainstream use.

For now, Dr Ekechi says, what early-pregnancy units can – or
should – do is to talk people through whether 'there are features
on the scan that are reassuring or, maybe, if there are features
that are not reassuring'. Though what is and isn't reassuring is, in
itself, far from clear-cut. Take a subchorionic haematoma, for
example, which is thought to be the most common cause of
bleeding in early pregnancy, accounting for around one in ten
cases. Although the discovery of a haematoma – which Dr
Ekechi describes as being rather like a 'bruise' where the baby
has implanted – can at least offer an alternative explanation for
where the bleeding is coming from, other than an imminent
miscarriage, it does not rule out the possibility of miscarriage
altogether. And it's unclear whether having a haematoma
reduces or raises your risk overall. While some large studies have
suggested the presence of a bleed like this can increase the risk
of miscarriage (almost two-fold, according to one large review
of evidence based on data from 70,000 women[4]) others, such as
a 2020 study of more than 1,000 IVF pregnancies, have concluded that it makes no difference to the live-birth rate.[5]

'We've been trying to understand whether the presence of a
haematoma automatically means that a miscarriage is occurring –
and we haven't actually found a correlation in that regard,'

confirms Dr Ekechi. 'Many women come with a small sub-chorionic haematoma in early pregnancy and that pregnancy continues to develop and the haematoma is absorbed over time.' Adding still more confusion, some women seem to have haematomas – and healthy pregnancies – but don't bleed at all.*

What else could give a clue as to what your bleeding means? A baby the right size for the estimated gestational age can be reassuring. Growth in the earliest weeks of pregnancy is very rapid, and, as such, trained professionals can date the pregnancy not only according to the week of gestation but to the day (e.g., six weeks plus one) using a metric known as 'crown-rump length'. This precise schema of measurements was developed by one of the pioneers of pregnancy ultrasound, Hugh Robinson, in 1973, and has been used almost unchanged ever since. (Yes, we had put a man on the moon before we routinely monitored what happens inside a woman's womb in pregnancy – let alone begun to map out and make sense of what we saw.) Generally, if what medics can see on-screen doesn't quite match up with where the pregnancy should be, according to the date of a woman's last period, it flags that all may not be well. However, doctors will often want to rule out the possibility someone has 'got their dates wrong' and is, in fact, less far along than they thought, by waiting for a follow-up scan to see if things progress normally. (Of course, if you have been trying to conceive for a while, diligently tracking your cycles, body temperature and other fertility signs to predict ovulation, the idea that you would have your period dates wrong, or have ovulated a week later than you'd estimated, can feel almost laughable.)

In 2020, American researchers suggested that other key

---

* If it feels like we should know and understand more about what's believed to be the cause of more than one in ten cases of first-trimester bleeding, consider this: the very existence of subchorionic haematomas only became known to doctors in 1981, when they were described for the first time in the *British Journal of Obstetrics and Gynaecology*.

measurements taken during ultrasound scans might be better able to identify whether a pregnancy would ultimately prove non-viable – and at an earlier point. After monitoring 252 pregnancies, of which 61 ended in loss, taking various measurements from weekly ultrasound scans at between six and ten weeks gestation, they concluded that a smaller gestational sac than normal or an abnormally sized yolk sac (this is part of the embryo, and the first structure visible on an ultrasound) 'reliably predicted pregnancy loss'. 'In pregnancies destined to be lost, different ultrasound markers became abnormal at least one week before the loss,' the study authors explained in the journal *Scientific Reports*.[6] The yolk-sac measurements were the most reliably predictive, they found. All the pregnancies with a larger-than-normal yolk sac ended in a miscarriage by ten weeks, for example. Although it's not known for sure, one possible explanation is that a larger yolk sac indicates a chromosomally abnormal embryo. While the findings from this small study would need repeating, the authors suggested that they could be used to change current practice and the way women are counselled during early pregnancy. 'If these parameters [the yolk-sac and gestational-sac sizes] are normal at six weeks, the pregnancy will likely continue beyond the first trimester,' they said. Likewise, the absence of any abdominal pain can be an encouraging sign, according to Professor Regan. 'It is only when abdominal pains follow that the process starts to move in the direction of inevitability,' she suggests in her book *Miscarriage: What Every Woman Needs to Know*.

Perhaps the most obviously reassuring sign, for medics and expectant parents alike, is seeing a heartbeat on an early scan. Intuitively, this *feels* like it has to be a good sign. In our first pregnancy, we were told the risk of miscarriage was 'next to nothing' after seeing a heartbeat at six weeks. The breeziness with which this verdict was delivered – and the ease with which I believed it – has haunted me ever since.

There is, though, more than a grain of truth in the idea that the miscarriage risk drops once a heartbeat is seen. An NHS patient information leaflet from 2016 estimates that 'in the presence of a heartbeat there is an 85 per cent to 97 per cent chance of your pregnancy continuing'. If you're having an otherwise low-risk pregnancy – so, not a multiple pregnancy, not an IVF pregnancy, you're not over thirty-five or under seventeen, or with any serious underlying health conditions or a high BMI – some medical textbooks suggest the chance of an ongoing pregnancy is more like 97 or 98 per cent. This is reassuring – but much less so if you've been in that unlucky 2 or 3 per cent before.

'If you see a foetal heartbeat, it means that certain checkpoints or developmental milestones have been achieved,' explains Professor Nick Macklon, of the London Women's Clinic. 'And I used to advise patients – still do actually – that if you see a foetal heartbeat, there's probably more than a 90 per cent chance it's going to carry on. As soon as I say that, you can see their massive relief and joy.' It's not just the presence of the foetal heartbeat that's important, he adds, it's the speed. A slower heart rate than normal for the gestational age can be a sign a pregnancy is struggling – though it's still not considered a wholly reliable predictor of miscarriage.

Although the presence of a heartbeat is 'definitely a positive sign', Professor Macklon reflects, 'there probably is room for more caution among people like me when we see it.' Dr Ekechi agrees: 'The risk of miscarriage does drop – but it doesn't drop to zero. And I think people forget that. That's why it's important to say what early-pregnancy units can do – and, unfortunately, what we can't yet do.' She adds: 'It's a difficult conversation', especially in a society where, in general, there is 'reduced appetite' for uncertainty – to the point where doctors themselves may not always make clear the true extent of what they can't be sure of.

In my own experience, these conversations can be rushed, and the information you are offered impersonal and imprecise.

And for all that the invocation of the word 'miscarriage' is alarming, there is a jarringly relaxed attitude towards pregnancy bleeding. Take this, from one leaflet produced by an NHS hospital in 2018: 'we hope that your scan will reassure you that your pregnancy is continuing. Normally your bleeding should become lighter and eventually stop and will not have harmed your baby in any way.'[7] Or this, from an article published by a US health-insurance company: 'If it's happening to you, don't worry – everything is probably fine.'[8] Or this from *What to Expect When You're Expecting* about women who experience bleeding in early pregnancy: 'most go on to have a perfectly healthy pregnancy and baby'.[9] Perhaps worst of all is a video I stumble across on the NHS's advice website. 'Usually, it's absolutely fine when you've had any light bleeding early in the pregnancy, but do always remember to go and get it checked out either with your midwife or with your GP,' a uniformed midwife calmly explains to camera. Miscarriage and ectopic pregnancy are mentioned in the video, but only as serious events that may happen 'occasionally'. The video is bookended with stock footage of a pink, gurgling baby. I feel slightly nauseated watching it. My blood seems to run alternately cold and boiling. I do not find it remotely reassuring. I find it misleading.

To me, this is the same lack of specificity, even wilful evasiveness, that's at work when detailed miscarriage information is left out of antenatal leaflets and pregnancy handbooks, or when women are told that 'the majority', 'most', or 'almost all' miscarriages happen because there is something intractably wrong with the embryo, when in fact it could be that as many as half of lost pregnancies are genetically viable. Perhaps these elisions and half-truths come from the same well-intentioned place, trying to minimize distress – *It wasn't your fault, It will all be fine* – but such information gaps can end up doing the opposite. At the very least, it seems logically inconsistent to hand women leaflets titled 'Threatened Miscarriage' while also insisting that everything will 'almost always' be OK.

Perhaps it's this confused approach that explains why I'm reluctant to seek medical attention just yet. As much as I know that any bleeding in pregnancy should always be flagged with a healthcare professional, I also know that the most pressing danger associated with early bleeding (an ectopic pregnancy, which can be life-threatening) has already been ruled out in our case, thanks to the seven-week scan we had, almost two weeks ago now.

And if I am indeed going to have a fifth miscarriage, we'll want it to be handled by our clinic, rather than the local hospital, so that we have the best possible hope of getting further slivers of information to help us work out what might be going on. In short, to do anything but wait feels like a huge waste of everyone's time and energy. The intense drive I felt just days ago, propelling me to ask my doctors for something – anything – new to try has evaporated into grim acceptance once more. For now, then, Dan and I settle for *que sera, sera*. We pretend we are sanguine. We pretend we know how we will cope with a fifth disappointment. I add sanitary pads to the weekly shop, along with my favourite bottle of wine and Dan's preferred cider, though we do not open them yet. 'To Be Drunk in Case of a Miscarriage,' we joke. Our main discussion centres around logistics – specifically: what we will do if I need surgery to remove the pregnancy, as I've had to have before. In the week I start bleeding, we are also in the death-throes of a protracted attempt to move house. If it goes ahead, we will be relocating 200 miles away two days after the appointment at which we fully expect a miscarriage will be diagnosed.

We have been trying to move since the summer, and it is now the first week in December. Relocating away from London is the latest in a chain of events set in motion by finding out there was no obvious reason for our miscarriages. First, just before our fourth pregnancy, I'd decided to go freelance and handed in my notice. I had a job on a newspaper, which I loved, but which, in truth, I had outgrown. More than anything, I wanted to be in control of my own time. And I wanted a life that had a little more space in it. There were things I felt I should be doing ahead of another pregnancy: counselling, acupuncture, perhaps more yoga. There was also a question, still percolating, as to whether we should seek out more tests and treatment privately, which would all take time and bandwidth. Above all, I'd been working, flat out, since graduation, in the hope of reaching a secure place in my journalism career in time to start a family. I'd never – not really – stopped to consider what I actually wanted my life to look like. I took the jobs I was offered. I did as I was told, arrived on time, stayed late, and dressed the part. I'd worked nightshifts and weekends; bank holidays and Christmases. It had felt like success at the time – at least some of the time, anyway. But, nearly a decade on, I was left wondering what it had all been for.

Suddenly, it felt naive to be treading water at work for the sake of qualifying for twelve weeks of maternity pay. Because, what if I never needed it? For the first time, I sat and thought about what I really wanted, other than a baby. If Dan and I weren't going to float happily with the crowd, having children at roughly similar times to our friends, slipping seamlessly into the primary-coloured world of soft-play, our weekends filling up with kids' parties and swimming lessons, what were we going to do? Who would we be, if not parents?

We decided to start with *where* we would be. Once we'd worked out that I could earn enough money freelancing, we had more options. Dan and I may have been tired of London, but we were not tired of life – we wanted more of it. I yearned for something bigger, in a way that had nothing to do with square-footage.

We stopped looking at catchment areas. We stopped looking at practical 'family' houses. I started dreaming of cottages, cow parsley, and drystone walls. Which is how we'd found a perfectly impractical house, clinging on to the hem of a village, where Greater Manchester rolls away into the Peak District. When I think of this new house, and us in it, I don't picture a nursery. I think about the friends we can host when they need a weekend away from the city. I think about noisy dinners around a long, farmhouse table. I think of linen dried by clean air and sweet peas growing by the door. I think of reading by the fire in winter and having breakfast outside in summer. I want to really *live* in this next house, instead of just commuting to and from it. It's not that we've made our peace with a child-free future, exactly. Deep down, the move represents more a sort of provocation to the universe: look, here we are, forging ahead, making other plans. After all, isn't that when real life is supposed to happen? Indeed, when it looked like the sale would collapse, I reminded myself that it was far better this way round. I was still pregnant. Now, though, it is looking increasingly like both things are going to slip away from us.

Then, one Friday, a few days after I'd started to bleed, we learn that the sale has gone through. The bleeding doesn't stop, but it doesn't get worse either.

We stick with our plan to hold our breath until the Wednesday appointment. I feel oddly removed from what is, or isn't, happening, displaced from my own body. It is so different from the first time I saw unwanted blood, during my first pregnancy.

Dan and I had been away for the weekend for a wedding and were finally back in the hotel room after a long day. When I'd gone to the loo, the toilet paper came away streaked with pink slime. I checked the toilet bowl . . . Also pink. This was not happening, I thought. It couldn't be happening – not now. I had only just told Mum, at her birthday dinner, that she was going to be a granny. After a panicked google, rather than travel straight to the local hospital, Dan and I decided to wait until morning. There was a single sentence during our internet search I will never forget reading: '*Once a miscarriage has started, it cannot normally be prevented.*' But there were other words, too – more reassuring ones: '*Bleeding is really common in early pregnancy.*' '*It's not always a sign of miscarriage.*' '*It's probably nothing.*'

We bailed on the post-wedding, hangover brunch and headed to the nearest early-pregnancy unit, which was open at weekends – a stroke of luck I didn't fully appreciate at the time; most EPUs have astonishingly limited opening hours.* Still, they couldn't scan me then and there – being a Sunday, there wasn't anyone in to do it – but they took a blood test and felt my abdomen to check I was not in pain, which could indicate an ectopic pregnancy. Because we were out-of-towners, they arranged for someone to call me in the morning with the blood test results; if these suggested an ongoing, viable pregnancy, they would refer me for a scan closer to home. And the next day, we found ourselves walking out of the maternity ward at our local hospital, with a leaflet titled 'Threatened Miscarriage' and our baby's perfect, flickering heartbeat imprinted in our minds. A false alarm. 'A scare,' we tell the few friends and family who know. 'All fine.' Except, of course, it wasn't, in the end.

---

* While it's hard to say definitively, as a complete list of the number of early-pregnancy units in the UK doesn't appear to be kept, fewer than twenty out of at least 200 units open seven days a week, according to a – now rather old – NHS report. This is despite seven-day services being recommended by the health watchdog NICE. Of those that do operate seven days a week, many open only for a very limited amount of time per day. I could find only three early-pregnancy units in the UK that opened all hours, seven days a week. Within 100 miles of London, I couldn't find even one. Instead, most EPUs tend to keep strict weekday office hours. In some cases, they open only for a couple of hours a day, or on a couple of set days per week. Many do not accept walk-ins, only GP referrals. To point out the obvious, miscarriages do not keep tidy office hours, only happening between 9 a.m. and 5 p.m., Monday to Friday.

When it comes to threatened miscarriage, we have 'no social or cultural scripts in which to understand this experience', the medical historian Rosemary Elliot has noted. Elliot's own first encounter with miscarriage was the threat of one, by way of unpromising blood test results, pain and a suspected ectopic, which all turned out to be OK. 'The explanation was that the blood test results were wrongly recorded,' she writes. 'My relief that my pregnancy was in fact continuing overrode any sense of annoyance at the ten-day uncertainty around that fact. It seemed ungrateful to complain, when the outcome was a continuing pregnancy and a healthy baby.'[10]

But even when the threat of miscarriage dissipates, and a pregnancy progresses, bleeding early on is not necessarily without consequence. One comprehensive review of the evidence found a link between threatened miscarriage and further complications such as an increased risk of bleeding in the second and third trimesters, low birth-weights, early labour (before thirty-seven weeks) and very early labour (before thirty-four weeks), although the authors did say that some of the evidence was from small, imperfect studies and larger trials were needed (again, this is a depressingly recurring theme in this area of medicine).[11] Other research has suggested that after early vaginal bleeding in pregnancy, the risk of a second-trimester miscarriage increases (although the overall risk remains low) from 1.2 per cent, if someone has no bleeding, to 2.2 per cent.[12]

Against this conflicting, confusing landscape, it's little wonder the internet pulls you in like an irresistible force. I search and I search and I search – reading everything, believing nothing. I find one study, from 2009, that attempted to unravel the significance of bleeding in early pregnancy when a miscarriage does not follow within several days – does this mean a miscarriage is still more likely than not to be looming in the future? The authors of the trial tried to answer this question by excluding from their results any episodes of bleeding that happened

four days or fewer before a miscarriage was subsequently confirmed. What they concluded from this data-set – when any
bleeding could be considered distinct from the miscarriage
'main event', so to speak – was that spotting (which meant only
noticing blood when someone wiped) and light bleeding
(which meant lighter than someone's normal, menstrual bleeding) was not associated with any increased risk of loss,
particularly when it did not last more than one or two days.
However, when a bleeding episode was heavier, with at least
one day of bleeding that was heavier than someone's normal
period, the risk of miscarriage was three times higher than for
women who have no bleeding.[13]

I spend a lot of time parsing my symptoms for meaning. But
on almost every metric, I can make the case to myself both
ways: my bleeding is not particularly heavy, just spots, requiring a thin pantyliner. But it has gone on for almost a week now.
I don't have any pain. The measurements at our previous scan
put the pregnancy a couple of days behind where I thought I
was. I feel sick and exhausted, but no more so than in my previous pregnancies. I have not actually thrown up, not even
once. Then there is the confounding – and entirely unscientific –
factor of the house sale. I simply cannot believe we will get so
lucky as to have both things work out.

I barely sleep the night before the scheduled scan. My mum
comes with us to the hospital for moral support and also so
that, if things go badly, I won't have to be on my own if Dan
has to go back to work after the appointment. While we wait,
she manages to keep up a steady stream of one-sided conversation about her cycling, her knitting, and the roadworks on the
A14. I know what she's doing, trying valiantly to keep us distracted. But the only words my brain has space for are the ones
I am convinced I am about to hear for a fifth time: *I'm so sorry,
there is no heartbeat.*

When we're finally called in for the scan, I explain to the

sonographer that I am anxious. I stammer out our history and that I've been bleeding. We're in the same room we were in the last time I found out I'd miscarried. I try not to look at the print on the wall, a red heart printed in swirly faux-brushstrokes. I try not to think what I thought back then, too: how fucking inappropriate that picture is. A heart, for when there is no heartbeat. I lie down on the bed and unbutton my jeans, exposing a slice of pale, soft stomach. Dan holds my hand, jaw clenched, staring straight ahead. Mum sits on the other side of him, silent now. I am braced for the words: *So sorry. So sorry* . . . Except they don't come. The sonographer is telling us that everything looks fine. She is turning the screen towards us – towards us, not away – and she is pointing out the flickering heartbeat. It's still there.

'You're nine weeks and one day,' she says, smiling. 'Everything looks great.'

The kidney-bean shape on the screen is moving, jiggling. Then it swims before my eyes. I am crying. I suddenly feel like I need sugar. A cup of hot, sweet tea, perhaps. I was not prepared for this. I apologize for crying. And then I laugh, high on relief. And then I apologize again.

'I'm sorry, it's just . . . I'm just . . . I don't know what to . . .' Of all the scenarios that played out in my head in the waiting room, this, I realize, was not one of them.

'Would you like to take a picture of the screen?' the sonographer prompts gently. I hesitate. I would like that, more than anything. But I daren't. Not yet. I shake my head.

'No, it's OK . . . I . . .'

Mum steps in. '*I'll* take a picture,' she says. 'You might decide you want it . . . later.'

And so I let her. I let her carry this small but significant piece of hope for me, for now.

5

'She doesn't carry well'

(December 2019 – 10 weeks pregnant)

The day after the scan, the movers arrive and pack everything we own into boxes with disturbing efficiency. Once it's all taken away, ready for transit the following day, I hoover the empty rooms, removing the last traces of dust and cat hair, until the only evidence of our life here is the network of furrows in the carpet left by our bookcases, tables, and beds. Dan and I spend the night in a cheap hotel. In the morning, we hand over our keys and drive north: two tired humans, three confused cats, and one foetus, as it can now be officially categorized.*

As we do all this, a referral from our GP is making its way between two NHS fax machines in an attempt to arrange our next appointments, back in standard antenatal care, having graduated from the recurrent-miscarriage clinic. The thought of beginning again with unfamiliar midwives and another

---

* Clinically speaking, a developing pregnancy is considered an embryo until week eight, and after that it's a foetus.

hospital feels like both a clean slate and a precipice. We've been in the new house exactly a week when the 'booking-in' appointment happens. Our new postcode, when I'm asked for it at reception, is still a foreign word on my tongue.

The appointment doesn't get off to a good start. The midwife, young with long, straight hair and wide, round eyes, comes into the room and announces brightly that she's not read our notes yet, then tells me that I look like one of the Kardashians.

'You know, the little one.'

'I'm afraid I don't watch it,' I say primly, taken aback more than anything. It's true, I don't know which Kardashian she means, but the way I reply makes it sound as though I am the kind of person whose only indulgences are rereading *Middlemarch* and growing kale. In fact, I have watched more than my fair share of reality television. But I cannot access the relevant memories and parts of myself in this moment. Humour, playfulness, small talk – they are all locked away for safekeeping. I am clamped shut like a bud against frost. Later, I will feel guilty, but for now I am simply, coldly furious at her failure to read the room. Dan squeezes my hand. I know he feels it, too. I also know he will find a way to make a joke about it later.

This is not who I am, I want to tell the wide-eyed midwife. Not really. I want to explain; I want to tell her how this pregnancy, and the miscarriages before it, have unwritten every story I used to believe about myself and my own body. How it has undermined the strength, predictability, and resilience that I always took for granted. I am almost obnoxiously healthy: I heal fast and get over bugs quickly. My periods are well-behaved and tidy. I rarely get headaches and I don't feel the cold. I like to run, lift weights, and dig in the garden. I am not, on the whole, a precious person. But perhaps that's because I never had a reason to be until now. Before, I never stopped to consider how lucky I was in my own body, how much space this

allowed for other things. I want to tell the midwife that this is
not the kind of pregnancy I thought I'd be having. At one
point, I'd assumed it would be easy and rather fun. I could tell
her how, in the past, I was secretly a little scornful of those who
made heavy weather out of being pregnant, fussing about their
exposure to 'toxins' or the prospect of a late night. When it came
to my turn, I'd always imagined I'd be different – practical,
undemanding. Just me, only pregnant. Pride, as they say, comes
before a fall.

Blame, failure, and a notion of female weakness – reproductive
unfitness – is inherent in the word 'miscarriage'. In 2018, an
Instagram post by the actor James Van Der Beek went viral after
he shared his and his wife Kimberley's experience of multiple
miscarriages and stated that 'we need a new word for it'. '"Miscarriage", in an insidious way, suggests fault for the mother – as
if she dropped something, or failed to "carry",' he wrote. In
many languages, miscarriage is often described 'in terms of falling', according to the medical anthropologist Dr Susie Kilshaw,
a principal research fellow at UCL whose work focuses on fertility and reproductive loss. For example, 'in Arabic, miscarriage is
referred to as *isqat* or *tasqeet*, both originating from *saqat* (to miscarry), which means to "drop something from up to down",' she
writes.[1] In British Sign Language, the gesture to convey a miscarried pregnancy is to hold both hands against your chest and
then to flick them down and away. In French, the word for miscarriage is *fausse-couche*, a conjunction that translates roughly as
'wrong' or 'false' childbirth. What's more, in French you do not
'have' a miscarriage, you *faire une fausse-couche* – the verb *faire*
meaning 'to do' or 'to make'. It is not something that merely
happens to you; it is something your body actively *does*. Alongside
the blame – in English, at least – the word miscarriage is also suf-
fused with a sense of something that should never have happened
in the first place, perhaps because of its other common usage, in

the context of the law: a miscarriage of justice, with all its con-
notations of mistake and misunderstanding. Indeed, in previous
centuries, women referred to a suspected miscarriage as a 'mis-
hap', a 'miss', a 'slip', or an 'accident'. In this single word, then –
miscarriage – we are, at once, blamed for not holding on tighter to
the pregnancy and shrugged at as if we should have known all
along that this wasn't the right one. Even all-encompassing terms
such as 'pregnancy loss' or 'baby loss' – increasingly preferred
today for their apparent softness and ability to unite women who
have had miscarriages, ectopic pregnancies, unsuccessful IVF
transfers, terminations for medical reasons, stillbirths, or babies
who died in infancy – are not free from notions of self-blame.
Although I often express it this way, I didn't 'lose' my baby. I did
not absent-mindedly forget to keep being pregnant. I did not
misplace it or leave it behind somewhere. I was not careless. It
died. The small lifeform inside me stopped living.

No wonder we have such a scrambled picture of cause and
effect. Perhaps the first barrier to true understanding of miscarriage is a linguistic one. Because, for all that some of the UK's
best specialists can tell me, following the best available evidence, there is no inherent weakness or fallibility in my body
that should hinder its ability to carry a baby. Yet, all the same,
I can't shake the feeling that pregnancy is something I am just
not very good at. I once heard a female relative say, many years
ago, of someone else: 'She doesn't carry well.' It's a damning
prognosis I can't help feeling applies to me now, too.

The midwife is making her way through her set questions
with cheerful alacrity, ticking boxes and jotting down our
answers in the green, hole-punched pamphlet that will become
my maternity notes for as long as this pregnancy lasts. We get to
the section of the form that asks about previous pregnancies.

'And . . . do you know . . . why – why that miscarriage, err,
happened?' the midwife asks, frowning just a little.

I tell her no. Her face falls. It falls further and further as we progress through the four pregnancies and everything we don't know. By the end, I feel vaguely guilty for putting *her* through this. I wonder at how much of a surprise this all seems to be to her. There's the slightest uptick of astonishment in her voice as she asks us: 'You didn't find out a reason for that one, either?'

Perhaps she was looking at Dan and me and thinking that the frequently cited risk factors didn't apply either. We are non-smokers, we are both under thirty-five (I was thirty at the time of my first miscarriage), we are both within what the medical establishment considers to be a healthy range for weight.

Along with your smoking status, your age, and your weight, the NHS also warns that drinking alcohol or 'lots' of caffeine while pregnant can also increase your risk of a miscarriage. It feels confusing, to put it mildly, when you are so often told 'it's nothing you did' after a miscarriage, only to be presented with a list of things that relate to what you might have done – or that you can't control, like your age. How much nicer it would be if someone first handed you a reassuring list of what isn't to blame. For example, it wasn't because you had a previous ter- mination. It isn't caused by running, having sex, or because you lifted something heavy that one time. It isn't caused by sitting at a computer all day for work *or* by standing up all day for work. It also won't be down to the glass of wine you had before you knew you were pregnant. None of these things increase your risk.* There's evidence to show as much. Not that we

---

* In the earliest weeks of pregnancy, an embryo actually forms in a protected 'hypoxic' environment – hypoxic means free from oxygen. Oxygen in the mater- nal bloodstream can have 'free radicals' – highly reactive molecules – that could potentially cause a pregnancy to implant and develop abnormally. So, up until about five weeks, an embryo is protected accordingly. In other words, it doesn't yet need or take much of its blood supply from you at all. It is effectively sealed off in its own little bubble, largely indifferent to what is or isn't circulating in your blood. However, this is a nuance that seems to be neglected by health messaging, in our haste to reduce harm that can be caused by heavy drinking and drug use later on in pregnancy.

seem to have absorbed this into our wider culture and how we think about miscarriage.

Age, on the other hand, is prominent in the public imagination when it comes to having babies. The tired trope of the ticking biological clock looms large, especially for women. While the popularized notion that fertility 'falls off a cliff' after the age of thirty-five is not quite as clear-cut as many women have been made to believe,[*] when it comes to miscarriage rates, the stark reality is that the risk does increase, the older you are. This is thought to be down to the natural decline in egg-cell quality over time. This means the eggs become more fragile with age and more prone to developing chromosomal errors as each egg reaches maturity before fertilization. According to one of the papers on miscarriage published in the *Lancet* series in 2021,[2] which reviewed all the available, relevant data, the risk of trisomy 16 (three copies of chromosome pair 16 and the most common cause of miscarriage) rises 'linearly' between the ages of twenty and forty, whereas the risk of other trisomies that can lead to miscarriage rises more sharply from 'around the age of thirty-five'. Previous research in which scientists were able to genetically analyse lost pregnancies found that as many as 80 per cent of miscarriages in women over forty had a chromosomal abnormality of some kind.[3] The good news, buried within that unpromising statistic, is that if you are over forty and can bear to keep going until you alight on a genetically 'normal' pregnancy,

---

[*] This idea was exploded in a now much-referenced 2013 piece for the *Atlantic* by the psychologist and researcher Jean M. Twenge. As Twenge discovered, 'the widely cited statistic that one in three women aged 35 to 39 will not be pregnant after a year of trying' does not come from contemporary data, but from French birth records from 1670 to 1830. 'In other words, millions of women are being told when to get pregnant based on statistics from a time before electricity, antibiotics, or fertility treatment,' she writes, going on to point out that the few available studies that have looked at female age and natural fertility in modern cohorts are comparatively more optimistic.

the odds are there'll be no other reason it wouldn't be successful.*
Overall, though, the *Lancet* review concluded that female age has
a 'profound' effect on the risk of miscarriage, estimating that in
women between the ages of twenty and twenty-nine, the chance
is around 12 per cent (equating to slightly less than one in eight
pregnancies), rising to a 65 per cent risk by the time a woman is
forty-five (more than one in two).

Of course, immediately after a miscarriage, knowing the
difference that age makes does not feel all that helpful. It's
information that's potentially as dispiriting whether it applies
to you or not. On the one hand, your age is something you can
do nothing at all to modify. On the other, if time is on your
side – statistically, at least – it feels like no kind of explanation
at all. (And, in my case, makes you question whether this means
it's *more* likely there's something else 'wrong' with you.)

Sometimes, it feels like age is wielded as an excuse not to
learn or do more about miscarriage. But, conversely, if you are
smack bang in the prime of your reproductive years, and therefore statistically less likely to miscarry, the medical profession is
in no more of a rush to investigate what might be going on.
Sometimes, it feels like the foremost answer medicine has for
preventing miscarriage is to warn women not to 'leave it too
late'. And yet, despite recent calls for girls to be taught in school
or university about their short biological shelf life, or even suggestions that contraceptive pills should carry cigarette-box-style
warnings about declining fertility, the narrative that women
leave it too late because they are simply unaware is unconvin-
cing, at best. Studies have repeatedly found that the leading
reason women delay starting a family is not reluctance,
ignorance, or naivety, but not having found a suitable partner

---

* Indeed, the same study found that 75 per cent of women over forty did not miscarry in the first place.

yet.* In 2016, Danish researchers gave a cohort of (mostly female) university students a questionnaire to try to establish their attitudes towards parenthood and their knowledge about fertility. Three quarters of the female participants surveyed said that they ideally wanted their first child when they were between twenty-five and twenty-nine. Only 2 per cent stated that they wished to have their first child over the age of thirty-five. Sixty per cent said they wanted to have completed their families before they were thirty-five – suggesting that women are well aware of the constraints of biological time. Yet, curiously, this is not how the findings of this study were presented. The top line offered in the published paper was that '40 per cent of all respondents [i.e. men and women] intended to have their last child after the age of thirty-five years' and the level of fertility knowledge was 'of concern'.

Of course, something that often doesn't make it into public-health messaging is that a father's age increases the risk of miscarriage, too – the *Lancet* research series identified that if a man is over forty his partner has an increased risk of having a miscarriage, regardless of her age.† Yet while there are plenty of biologically plausible reasons that advancing male age would increase the risk of pregnancy loss, such as more genetic abnormalities in sperm cells, it is much less well studied – as researchers writing in the journal *Human Reproduction Update* in 2020 pointed out.[4] As yet, they also noted, there have been no studies at all looking at the relationship between the age of the male

---

* Such as one 2018 study led by a Yale University anthropologist, who interviewed women about the reasons they were freezing their eggs. Contrary to the persistent stereotype, 'partnership problems, not career planning' was the reason most women gave for pursuing egg-freezing.

† Older men do tend to have partners of a similar age, but the *Lancet* researchers adjusted their data to take into account confounding factors – meaning anything that might complicate the results other than what is being studied, such as the mother's age – and the age of the father was still found to make a difference to the risk of miscarriage.

partner and recurrent miscarriage. It's a sly kind of medical misogyny, this – one that props up an idea that women's bodies alone are responsible for the fate of a pregnancy.

What's more, contrary to a prevailing narrative that, when it comes to fertility, younger is always better, miscarriage risk is also higher in women under twenty. Why might this be, considering that the risk of chromosomal errors – presumed to be the most common cause of miscarriage – should be lowest in this group? That younger, as well as older, women seem to be slightly more likely to miscarry than women in their mid- to late twenties is something that one group of Norwegian researchers described as a 'curious finding' when it showed up in an analysis in 2019.[5] They theorized that it could be down to lifestyle differences or it could be an as-yet not fully understood 'effect of reproductive immaturity'. (This concept in itself – that someone of eighteen or nineteen might not yet be physically or medically best placed for pregnancy – flies against all kinds of deeply ingrained ideas about 'peak' fertility in a culture that routinely fetishizes and sexualizes very young women and girls.)

Of course, while miscarriage appears to be more likely in younger women – twenty being much younger than the average age for first-time motherhood in the UK, of 28.9 – it is rare to hear accounts of miscarriage from this life-stage, perhaps because it falls outside of the typical magazine narrative of unambiguous sadness at losing a much-wanted pregnancy, though it's not a given that a pregnancy to a nineteen- or twenty-year-old will be unplanned. And even in an unplanned pregnancy, it doesn't follow automatically that a miscarriage will be a source of relief. But these kinds of preconceptions further isolate those who miscarry at this age. 'Whilst I blamed myself and vigorously tried to work out what I had done wrong, my parents had a sense of relief about them,' writes one anonymous seventeen-year-old, who miscarried shortly after receiving an offer of a university place. 'I know that they were relieved because they wanted me to have a normal teenage life and not be tied down with the responsibility of a child, but I wish that they would understand that just as they wanted the best for me, I wanted the best for my child.'[6]

Taken together, here's another possible explanation for why we've allowed miscarriage to continue as such a poorly understood subject: it disproportionately, though not exclusively, affects women that society tacitly disapproves of: older mums, teen mums – and overweight mums. After age, weight is the next risk factor that figures prominently in health advice around miscarriage. The 2021 *Lancet* review concluded that the lowest risk of miscarriage is for people whose BMI falls within the healthy range of 18.5 to 24.9,[7] though an analysis of patient data from the St Mary's Hospital recurrent-miscarriage clinic in London (my clinic) found that an additional risk of miscarriage only significantly increases once someone's BMI is above 30 (classed as obese, as far as medicine is concerned). This 2012 study found that, among recurrent-miscarriage patients with no known cause for their losses, the risk of having another miscarriage was 59 per cent for women with a BMI of at least 30, compared with 44 per cent for those who had a 'normal' BMI.[8] Yet, unlike age, it's much less clear what exactly carrying more weight does to the body that would increase the risk. For instance, it's not known definitively whether excess weight increases the chance of a chromosomal abnormality or does something else that contributes to miscarriage, although one small study, published in 2010, did find that women with a BMI of over 25 were more likely to lose apparently 'healthy' pregnancies which didn't have any chromosome defects.[9] The authors pointed to things such as insulin resistance and the condition polycystic ovary syndrome (PCOS) – which incidentally makes weight loss much harder – as possible contributing factors that needed further research. Other scientists have suggested that the inflammatory chemicals secreted by fat stores can impact the behaviour of the womb lining in pregnancy and/or cause blood vessels to function abnormally, contributing to miscarriages.

Whenever studies find a link between weight and miscarriage risk, the take-home message is usually that patients should be counselled about the link and encouraged or supported to lose weight ahead of a subsequent pregnancy. While there is some – limited – evidence that women with a BMI over 30 who complete a six-month diet and exercise programme subsequently have a lower rate of miscarriage than those who do not complete it,[10] we are also increasingly coming around to the idea that losing weight is an infinitely more complicated calculus than 'eat less, move more'. Eating habits and body size are an entangled matrix of emotions, hormones, sleep, stress levels, and all kinds of social privilege (or lack thereof). 'Weight bias' has been shown to be prevalent in healthcare, with a tendency to attribute any and all health issues to someone's weight without due consideration. Combine this with the reflex to self-blame after a miscarriage, and you have a potently toxic combination.

Dr Sarah Bailey is a former midwife, a researcher, and now the lead nurse for recurrent-miscarriage care at University Hospital Southampton NHS Foundation Trust. She says that when it comes to discussing weight with miscarriage patients, 'you walk a very difficult line'. She tells me: 'You don't want people to think this is the reason they miscarried. But we need to let couples know about the importance of optimizing their lifestyle. We know that maternal weight is a contributory factor to miscarriage – but you have to be really tactful, supportive and compassionate when you give that information. I always say: "That won't be the reason you miscarried, but it could help you to have a successful pregnancy outcome in the future, if you try to optimize your weight,"' pointing out that it's as important to address a very low BMI as a high BMI. She adds that, for some, it can be a positive step 'because it gives them back a bit of control in a situation where they've otherwise got no control'. I understand this. Anything that gives you back some kind of agency feels worth a try. Yet the way information about these key risk factors – age and weight – is deployed is not politically neutral. We are frequently reminded that the women embarking on motherhood today are older and heavier than in previous generations. Scientists have known for a long time that both age and weight increase the risk of miscarriage. On the basis that all of these things are true, it's not unreasonable to wonder if this means more women than ever will be affected.* And yet this does not seem to have combined to make miscarriage a more pressing health priority. Instead, women are made both the problem and the solution; as if 'don't leave it too late' and 'lose weight' are enough. It reinforces a notion – already instinctive after pregnancy loss – that miscarriage is a matter of personal responsibility.

There are other potential contributing factors to miscarriage risk that are less well understood, such as genetics. Researchers based in Aberdeen, Scotland, have suggested that miscarriage and recurrent miscarriage appear to be more likely if someone has a family history of it.[11] This line of enquiry interests me because, in the wake of our losses, Dan and I discovered that, in both our families, we are not the only ones to have had multiple miscarriages – though, as is often the case, we did not know this until we spoke about our own. Yet it's not known precisely what level of family history is most relevant to your own chance of miscarriage – i.e., on which side of your family, or whether it has to be a first-degree relative or not. The team from Aberdeen also pointed out that there is an obvious potential for bias in their findings, in that those with their own history of miscarriage may be more likely to report a family

---

* Of course, without official national data on the number of miscarriages that happen, we have no way of knowing if this is, in fact, the case.

history. Certainly, it's been my experience that you're only likely to know about a family member's miscarriage once you let it be known that it happened to you, too. Hence social taboos around this subject reinforce the gaps in scientific knowledge – and the vicious cycle continues.

Then there is deeply unedifying evidence emerging that suggests race makes a significant difference to someone's chance of having a miscarriage. While we don't have detailed UK-specific data, the 2021 *Lancet* research series estimated that Black women have a 40 per cent higher risk compared with white women. As for why this should be: 'We don't know – is the short answer,' says Dr Christine Ekechi, a specialist in early pregnancy and also the spokesperson for racial equality for the UK's Royal College of Obstetricians and Gynaecologists. 'Black women may be over-represented in the groups that are high risk for miscarriage, for example certain conditions that can increase the risk, but I don't think that's necessarily the whole answer,' she continues. 'For some, there may be biological factors. For others there might be societal and structural factors. The only thing that links all Black women is the race that's been assigned to them by society. It's important, therefore, that we don't homogenize a whole group of people based on the colour of their skin. To try to create a solution based on that is not helpful without actually drilling down into what the answer is.'

Of course, she adds, that doesn't mean we don't need this information, or that we shouldn't collect this kind of data, but 'it's important, particularly when we look through the lens of race and see these differences, that we really understand it's less about the racial group of these women and more about us as a society. It's about how we live in racialized societies and how that impacts on health.' According to Dr Ekechi, without accounting for this complexity, 'collecting and describing racial differences only serves to traumatize a group of people by telling them they have poorer outcomes without getting to the nub of the issue'. What's more, as with age and weight, there's a risk that emphasizing the role of race ends up functioning as an implicit kind of blame – or, at best, falsely portrays Black women's losses as biologically inevitable. 'It can become a reason to dismiss it,' confirms Dr Ekechi.

Perhaps the fact that key risk factors do not apply in my case is why I've felt able to tell my story of an experience that is so often labelled taboo. I am neither too old nor too fat, nor do I have too much melanin in my skin cells, so that my losses can be explained away. Perhaps on some semi-conscious level I knew I would not be blamed by the outside world, even as I tried to find reasons to blame myself on the inside.

Once you have more than three miscarriages in a row, in the UK at least, you qualify for further investigation into the possible medical causes, beyond the catch-alls about chromosomal errors, age, weight, cigarettes and alcohol. Although, as Dr Sarah Bailey tells me, with not a little frustration, there is still 'quite a variation' in what you might be tested for. In general, NHS centres should look for a range of issues that affect blood-clotting, which can potentially be treated with different regimens of medication, and also for structural issues to do with the shape of the womb, such as a 'heart-shaped' uterus, a unicornuate uterus (where only one side of the womb has developed), or a septate uterus (where there's an extra bit of muscle dividing the womb space). These structural abnormalities, which women are born with, often go undiagnosed until they have a baby – or try to – and are, in fact, relatively common beyond the realm of recurrent-miscarriage patients (so much so, gynaecologist Professor Lesley Regan has said, 'I often find myself wondering whether they should be called "abnormalities".'[12]) For women who have late miscarriages, a common diagnosis is the abysmally named 'cervical incompetence' – a weak or weakened cervix – which means the entrance to the womb opens, without warning, far too early in pregnancy. There are surgical procedures for some anatomical causes of miscarriage, such as removing muscle that's dividing up the womb or having a supportive stitch during pregnancy, known as cervical cerclage.

The most common – and treatable – known cause of recurrent miscarriage is antiphospholipid syndrome, or APS, found in around 15 per cent of recurrent-miscarriage patients. It's sometimes referred to as a blood-clotting disorder, but technically it is an autoimmune condition in which an overactive immune system produces antibodies – known as antiphospholipid antibodies – which attack fat or 'lipid' molecules in the blood, causing it to clot too quickly. In pregnancy, this can cause tiny clots that limit the flow of blood to the baby, while the antibodies also attack the developing placenta. However, treatment with a combination of low-dose aspirin and injections of the blood-thinner heparin have been shown to drastically improve the chance of a successful pregnancy, with live-birth rates rising from around 10 per cent when the condition is untreated to closer to 70 per cent. APS is sometimes nicknamed 'sticky blood' syndrome or Hughes syndrome, after Professor Graham Hughes, the British rheumatologist who first described the condition comprehensively – a medical discovery that happened only as recently as 1983. In part, this came about thanks to research into people who'd had multiple pregnancy losses. APS is now considered to be a major autoimmune disease and a key cause of stroke, deep vein thrombosis, and migraine, as well as recurrent miscarriage. It affects men as well as women. It's thought to be behind one in six heart attacks that occur in people under fifty. Which makes you wonder what other life-changing diagnoses we might make with more research into why miscarriages happen.

Sometimes, though – often, in fact – all of these possible causes will be ruled out. Being told that there is no 'cause' for your repeated miscarriages feels like the floor has given out beneath you. It happened to us one cold, bright January morning, six months after our third miscarriage. I'd barely taken my coat off before the doctor started rattling off the things I had tested negative for: antiphospholipid antibodies, lupus anti-coagulant, factor V Leiden, prothrombin gene mutation . . .

'I know it doesn't feel like it, but this *is* good news,' he said.

Dan went back to work straight after the appointment and, for reasons I can't really explain, even to myself, I decided to take myself shopping rather than go home alone. And so I stood staring at the flat, grey shop frontages, willing my feet to unstick themselves from the pavement. *How could the answer be nothing?*

I ended up wandering around the beauty hall of one of London's more famous department stores. Again, for reasons I can't explain, I let myself be persuaded to try a new facial, which used 'medical-grade lasers' to remove pollution and dead skin cells from your pores. Upstairs in the treatment room, the form I was handed asked if I'd had any surgery in the last year. I wrote in tight, cramped letters that six months ago I'd had an operation to remove the remains of a pregnancy, under general anaesthetic. When I handed the clipboard back to the beautician, she didn't mention it. I wished that she would. As I lay back and felt the hot ping of the laser dotting across my forehead, it struck me how ridiculous this was; that this laser-facial is something humans have figured out how to do. How someone, somewhere, in a lab or the boardroom of a cosmetics conglomerate, has come up with this – a solution to a problem that barely needed solving – and yet no one can tell me why I can't carry a baby.

The cause-less state you find yourself in without a definitive explanation for your miscarriages can be a frightening, boundless space. All the recrimination you had once directed at yourself, which you had been able to put to one side while you waited for a concrete, medical answer, comes pouring back.

With no known cause, the list of possible *unknown* causes feels infinite. You are cut adrift in a horizon-less sea of rec-ommendations from women on Mumsnet, private doctors, herbalists, healers, nutritionists, and ever-more-expensive fertility supplements. After the disappointment of our own inconclusive results, I read a cult bestseller that promises to tell you how to improve the quality of your eggs. Much of its advice was about reducing your exposure to certain 'hormone-disrupting' chemicals. I stopped wearing nail varnish and perfume. I stopped heating up food in plastic and tried to avoid touching till receipts. I bought another book, based on trad-itional Chinese medicine. In a bid to keep my womb 'warm', I took to wearing socks and slippers at all times, avoided cold floors, and added ginger oil to my bath. I didn't know how much I believed in any of it, but I did it anyway – anything to quell the anxiety that I was to blame, somehow. Anything to ignore my deepest fear: that I am fundamentally inhospitable; unsuited to motherhood.

The idea that miscarriage is always an act of maternal rejec-tion is ideological rather than based on biological fact. Indeed, the opposite may be true – in some cases, miscarriage could be a sign of the body acting in a way that is *'super-*maternal', according to Professor Nick Macklon, of the London Women's Clinic. Work by scientists including Professor Macklon and Professor Jan Brosens, of the University of Warwick, has iden-tified something they called the 'endometrial bio-sensor', a mechanism that does not seem to function as well in women who have multiple miscarriages. 'For just a few days a month, the lining of the womb is in condition to sense the quality of the embryo and decide whether to invest in it – or not,' explains Professor Macklon. Macklon and Brosens had been looking at the way the embryo and the lining of the womb (the endome-trium) interacted by studying both tissue types in the lab. They'd expected to see a flurry of activity when the endometrial cells reacted positively to an embryo, accepting it, and producing lots more molecules that would enhance implantation. Instead, as often happens in science, they found the opposite of what they were looking for. 'An embryo didn't seem to have any effect on the endometrium, unless it was a poor embryo,' says Professor Macklon. 'In which case, what we noticed was that the womb tissue started producing *less* of the molecules required for implantation.' In fact, a poor-quality embryo seems to trigger a kind of stress-response. But in women with a history of recurrent miscarriage, this response doesn't happen – instead the cells only detect the poor-quality embryo further on into pregnancy, resulting in a known miscarriage. 'So they accept embryos that another woman wouldn't,' adds Professor Macklon, who estimates that this could be the case for a third of women with unexplained recurrent miscarriage. A clue that this might be what's going on is if someone conceives relatively quickly – like I do. Our first three miscarriages happened in the space of nine months. Our fourth pregnancy was conceived within two menstrual cycles. This fifth one took three.

It's an idea I find comforting. Indeed, Professor Macklon tells me that after they published the paper explaining this theory, in 2012, he got 'a lot of emails from women who were, in some ways, very relieved by this explanation'.* It's not that our bodies don't carry well – it's that they carry too readily, too generously. We take on the most hopeless cases, we never give

---

* There is, Professor Macklon believes, a parallel theory contained in this discovery for why women who do not conceive easily, and for whom embryos repeatedly do not implant when they try IVF. They are, if you like, at the opposite end of the spectrum when it comes to the way their endometrial bio-sensor behaves. It's not that they are inhospitable, incompetent, or failing (or any of the other unhelpful adjectives often applied in fertility prognoses), it is that their wombs have immaculately high standards; they are perfectionists. However, as yet, this is just a hypothesis and has not been confirmed in studies.

up, we don't know when to stop. This, then, is the other story I want to tell the midwife today. This is the story I want to believe about myself. It feels more in keeping with what I thought I knew about my enthusiastic, hardy body.

Yet, there is one inconvenient wrinkle in this hypothesis. If this is the explanation for our losses, then it means the progesterone – the prescription on which we've pinned so much hope so far – might not be doing very much after all. And I don't like that idea one bit. But I can find no grand, unifying theory of these two ways of explaining myself to myself; no wormhole between the two possible realities. The wide-eyed midwife waves us off with an appointment for our dating scan – sometimes called the twelve-week scan. This is it, the one we've been waiting for. For many people, it is the first scan they have – the first major pregnancy milestone. For people like us, it feels like the end of a marathon. It's set for 30 December. Seventeen days to go.

6

'In case something happens'

(December 2019 – 12 weeks pregnant)

In theory, there is plenty to distract us from the wait for the dating scan. We have a house full of boxes to unpack and Christmas to get through. Yet still time seems to move both too slowly and unaccountably fast. Sometimes it feels like meagre drops from a dripping tap, each hour squeezing itself out miserably, while at others it is meted out in nervous, twitchy dollops; days that blur into one. I like it best when we are busy, exploring our new life here: shopping for a new bed, then a sofa, tracking down a snow shovel and a real Christmas tree, stocking the chest freezer, road-testing local cafes, finding new walking routes. We revel in the fact that whenever we set out in the car from our new home, rather than being confronted by the M25, we are sent out over implausible hillside passes, down into the Derbyshire Dales, or through the hulking caves of Victorian viaducts. These are the times I like best; when I feel safest. When we are driving somewhere. When we have purpose. When our attention is drawn outwards towards the horizon.

Because it is so easily pulled inwards and down, otherwise. Christmas is a terrible time to be this kind of pregnant. Quite apart from the booze and the unpasteurized cheese, there are too many songs on the radio that seem to vocalize your innermost thoughts: a cartoonish, jingle-bell rendition of your longing. *Baby, please come home. All I want for Christmas is you, baby.* After a meal out with friends, I find I cannot stop crying as Dan drives us home. Our news is still a secret, but another of our group is nearing the end of her pregnancy. And I think it is this that sets me off. I am suddenly so tired. Tired of bracing for bad news. Tired of inspecting the gusset of my knickers every time I go to the loo. Tired of pretending to drink my wine, in case anyone asks an uncomfortable question. I so badly want what our friend has: to be visibly, publicly pregnant. To absent-mindedly trace my fingers over my bump as I stand in a chattering crowd. To answer questions about whether we know if we're having a boy or a girl. To not only be pregnant, but to be actively, openly expecting to have a baby. Because, I realize, I may be pregnant, but I am not expecting anything, except another miscarriage.

Dan and I use the house move as an excuse not to go anywhere over Christmas itself. We congratulate ourselves for not miscarrying on Christmas Eve, on Christmas Day, on Boxing Day. And then suddenly, somehow, it's the morning of the scan – the day before New Year's Eve. It feels like it has arrived painfully slowly and all at once. I don't feel ready. What if this is the last morning I get to wake up still pregnant? I dress carefully, choosing the same clothes I've worn to the previous two scans: black stretchy jeans, which now only just do up, an oversized, soft grey jumper, and several fine-chained gold necklaces. I reread the bumpf of leaflets from the hospital and see that if you want a copy of the scan photo you have to pay £5. Fleetingly, I debate where we could get some cash out on the way, but decide this would definitely be jinxing things. I can't actually imagine being in the position to need that money. I also can't imagine being the kind of person whose main preoccupation ahead of this scan is the photo, how many copies of the picture they'll need, or, perhaps, how they'll use the image in an announcement afterwards. A coy Facebook update? (*Look what's arriving in 2020!*) A grinning selfie with the scan picture? An elaborate visual gag involving a bun and an oven? No. I cannot transpose my and Dan's experience on to any of it. Increasingly, when I see other people doing these things, performing the rites of pregnancy in this way, it feels like watching the interactions of another species.

An enduring social convention is that you do not announce a pregnancy until after twelve weeks – the end of the first trimester. But if we didn't have this twelve-week 'rule', it would quickly become plainly, painfully obvious how common miscarriage is. Around 85 per cent of all miscarriages happen before twelve weeks, which means that because they happen in as-yet-unannounced pregnancies, the miscarriages often go untold too. The obvious irony, of course, is that, for many people, the reasoning behind not announcing any earlier is 'in case something happens'. Simultaneously, then, miscarriage is made central to the experience of early pregnancy and reinforced as a social taboo. Along with playing a significant part in keeping miscarriage undiscussed, the custom also sets up a hierarchy of pregnancy loss. Any miscarriage that happens before thirteen weeks, when the second trimester begins, is classified as an early miscarriage. 'But it doesn't *feel* early for the person who's been pregnant,' says Professor Jacky Boivin, a professor of health pyschology at Cardiff University who specializes in fertility and reproductive issues. 'The biology is one thing, but the psychology is another,' she tells me.

In some ways, for many women, the first trimester is when you feel *most* pregnant. You are tired in a way that sleep can't touch. You don't necessarily look pregnant, but your breasts can be painfully swollen and solid. There may be headaches, cramps, and constipation. You might be sick. You might feel faint. You might go for days with a mouth that won't stop watering, your saliva sour and metallic-tasting. You are hungry, constantly, but your taste buds are capricious. They need placating with nursery food – beige food. At any moment, things you previously thought were safe become vomit-inducing: milk on cereal, chocolate, chewing gum, peppermint tea. In some ways, this is precisely the time when you most need people to know you are pregnant; that, actually, you really do need to sit down on this train. Most people know that the first trimester comes with symptoms, and yet we've normalized not talking about them until afterwards – and only once it's safe to do so, in a happy, ongoing pregnancy. If you only know how the first trimester feels from pregnancies that ended in miscarriage, people really do not like it if you bring it up. They react very strangely. If you have no living children, and you begin a sentence 'Oh yes, I remember when I was pregnant', very often they will look at you as though you have slapped them or uttered a terrible curse. There is a sense that if you didn't make it out of the first trimester, what you had wasn't a pregnancy in the same way.

How did we arrive at this contradictory place, writing miscarriage into all our pregnancy rule books while effectively erasing it from everyday conversation? A notion that pregnancy – and the first trimester in particular – is a tentative and ambiguous time can be traced through many different cultures, according to the anthropologist Dr Susie Kilshaw. In Urdu and Punjabi, the early months of pregnancy are the *kuche maheene* or 'raw months', conveying a sense that it is tender and easily injured. The traditional Jewish response to a pregnancy announcement, in Hebrew, is not *Mazel tov* (congratulations) but *B'sha'ah tovah*, which literally means 'at a good hour' and confers both a wish that all will unfold well and the promise of congratulations in due course. And, of course, it's now an accepted medical fact that the risk of pregnancy loss is highest in the first trimester.

In terms of biological milestones, by the end of the first

trimester, the bones, muscles and organs of the body have formed. It's also around this time – between ten and twelve weeks – that the placenta has developed enough to take over as the main factory for producing key pregnancy-supporting hormones, such as progesterone. Up until this point, progesterone is produced by the corpus luteum (the cell structure that forms in the place where an egg is released from, in the ovary). The developing embryo gets its nutrition from a separate structure, the yolk sac, rather than from the mother's bloodstream. By the start of the second trimester, however, the complex matrix of blood vessels, immune cells, stem cells, and muscle cells that make up the placenta has matured enough to be able to function in the way most of us understand it to in pregnancy: it nourishes the growing foetus from the mother's blood, filters out potentially harmful particles, such as some viruses and bacteria, and carries away the baby's waste products. The fact that, during the first trimester, you are effectively growing a whole new organ from scratch is the explanation sometimes given for why you feel so tired during this time. How the placenta develops – or not – is believed to be critical to whether a pregnancy implants successfully in the first place and whether it continues or is miscarried. It is also believed that less serious defects in how the placenta constructs itself contribute to pre-eclampsia and foetal growth restriction later on in pregnancy. Yet, despite its importance, 'the placenta remains one of the least understood human organs', as a team of researchers from New Zealand put it in 2018.[1] The scientists were trying to delineate exactly how the cells of the placenta behave, develop, and evolve from the very earliest days of pregnancy. However, they said, there are still major gaps in our knowledge: whole cell groups whose origin story we do not know – we know they exist, but we don't know where they came from.*

---

* Again, what we do know, the researchers added, we know mainly thanks to 'snapshots' provided by tissue samples collected in historical – now unrepeatable

It makes sense that our ideas about when it is 'safe' to announce a pregnancy would coincide with a defining stage in its development, such as the point at which the placenta takes over. And yet, the idea that the risk of miscarriage suddenly drops away at twelve weeks isn't quite right, either. Rather than the end of the first trimester representing some kind of bright line, studies have suggested that the risk of pregnancy loss actually falls incrementally, week on week.[2] In other words, there isn't a miscarriage cliff edge, and, in fact, the most significant drop in risk may come at an earlier point than twelve weeks.

According to obstetrician and researcher Professor Nick Macklon, as well as the womb lining having a way of differentiating between viable and non-viable embryos around the time of implantation – the 'endometrial bio-sensor', as it's been called – the womb lining may perform multiple status checks like this throughout early pregnancy to ensure all is developing as it should, determining whether the body continues to invest in the pregnancy or not. 'We now think there isn't just one checkpoint, there are probably three or four, up to about twelve or thirteen weeks,' he tells me. In some cases of miscarriage, if a pregnancy is miscarried at, say, nine weeks, 'it could be a checkpoint kicking in appropriately – upsettingly, but appropriately', Professor Macklon explains. 'The challenge for us in our field is to differentiate those miscarriages from the ones where it shouldn't have kicked in.' This, he says, is 'a key research need'. That there might be subtle variations in the pathology of miscarriages at different points in early pregnancy is an idea that feels instinctively logical to me, familiar as I am with my own pattern of loss, knowing how our pregnancies

---

– studies, because it is so difficult to study in real time without interfering with an ongoing pregnancy, or even in the lab, due to strict rules around the age of embryos that can be kept.

seem to make it far enough to show signs of cardiac activity, before faltering and falling silent a week or two later.

But if it's not perfectly consistent with the biology, what else might have led us to the twelve-week rule?

In part, it may be a hangover from a time in the really-not-that-distant past when women had to wait for physical proof to confirm their pregnancy, in the form of multiple missed periods or even once they started to feel the baby move, which generally happens between sixteen and twenty weeks. While the hormone that indicates pregnancy, HCG, was identified in the 1920s, the first at-home pregnancy test only became available to buy in British pharmacies in 1971 (and, even then, Boots refused to stock it – only 'fast' women would require a fast test). In Joan Didion's novel *Play It As It Lays*, published in 1970 and set in the late 1960s, the protagonist, Maria, tries to obtain a 'rabbit test' to establish whether she is pregnant. The 'rabbit test' was a legitimate and surprisingly accurate scientific method at the time and involved injecting a live female rabbit with a woman's urine – if the rabbit, which was in due course killed and dissected, had ovulated (a consequence of the HCG hormone), it was taken as a positive result. A similar method developed by a British scientist, and also used throughout the 1940s, 1950s, and 1960s, used frogs, which would lay eggs if there was HCG in the injected urine sample. However, perhaps unsurprisingly, neither of these methods was routinely used, unless there was a pressing medical need to establish or rule out whether a woman was pregnant (such as a suspected tumour). While pregnancy testing was technically available on the NHS from the 1940s, it was not available on demand for most women – indeed, many GPs openly disapproved of what was considered 'social' or 'curiosity' testing as an unnecessary burden on the health service.[3]

Even once scientists found ways to test for pregnancy that didn't require the use of live animals, throughout the 1970s women still had to visit a doctor to request a pregnancy test – a process that involved mixing a sample of their urine with specially modified sheep's blood and monitoring how 'clumpy' the mixture became. The earliest DIY pregnancy test kits used a version of this same method, and therefore looked like miniature chemistry sets rather than the stick tests we recognize and take for granted today – these lateral-flow pregnancy tests didn't become available until 1988. That's just shy of two decades after the moon landings, for anyone keeping score. Essentially, for all but the most recent generations of childbearing women, twelve weeks probably represented the earliest opportunity to establish with any certainty that you were pregnant. It was only at this point that the possibility of a baby could start to solidify into something real.

Deep-rooted cultural ideas about when a pregnancy becomes 'real' may also play their part in sustaining the twelve-week rule. 'Different societies have different ideas about how you invest in a pregnancy and when that being becomes a social being,' Dr Kilshaw tells me. In early modern Europe, for example, a foetus wasn't confirmed as real or considered a person before 'quickening', when a baby's movements could be felt for the first time – this was believed to coincide with 'ensoulment', that is, when a foetus acquires its own soul. (In the Islamic tradition, too, there is a similar time-frame for ensoulment, which, according to the Hadith, takes place 120 days, or four months, after conception – around the time movements typically start.) As such, according to the historian Lara Freidenfelds, there were rarely legal sanctions against behaviour that caused harm to a pregnancy before this point, whether that was a woman taking remedies to 'bring on' her period or a physical attack on the woman that caused her to miscarry. Women who committed crimes were also not exempt from execution if they believed they were pregnant but had not yet experienced quickening.[4] Even as modern, professionalized medicine started to emerge, in eighteenth-century Europe anything expelled by the potentially pregnant body before the three-month mark was understood as a 'false conception' by doctors – merely an accumulation of blood or rogue tissue rather than anything approaching a living being.[5]

Today, despite our easy access to highly sensitive, reliable pregnancy tests, the first trimester can still be experienced as a surreal, liminal state. You know you are pregnant, but you may not fully connect with that knowledge. In some ways, it still doesn't feel real yet. (This disjointed state functions slightly differently in a pregnancy like mine: after multiple miscarriages you are hyper-aware that you are pregnant, but you do not necessarily associate it with actually having a baby.) Dr Kilshaw suggests that the point at which this often changes is the first ultrasound scan. Rather than waiting for foetal movements, for many parents-to-be around the world, this is the point at which you are offered proof of your pregnancy, beyond a blue cross or two pink lines on a test that only you have witnessed. And, in many pregnancies, this often happens at the end of the first trimester. The ritual of the so-called 'twelve-week scan' exists in the UK, Australia, New Zealand, Canada, Denmark, Sweden, Ireland, and France, among other countries. 'In some ways, [the scan] is a bringing-forward of when you understood you were pregnant and that there was a being inside of you,' Dr Kilshaw tells me. 'Today, we emphasize biomedicine's ability to visualize and see, and it's less about what a woman can feel.'

But this scan is not offered at the twelve-week mark because it somehow represents a turning point in terms of miscarriage risk or how likely it is that your pregnancy will continue from hereon in; it's a ritual that's evolved out of developments in routine screening for conditions such as Down's syndrome. It's also a much more recent ritual than we might think. We take it for granted now, but women in the UK only started to be offered a scan at this point in pregnancy in the early 2000s, following the work of Professor Kypros Nicolaides and others at

King's College Hospital, in London, who came up with what is now called the combined screening test. This involves looking at the results of a blood test and data points such as a mother's age, along with measuring the fluid at the back of a baby's neck from an ultrasound scan in order to calculate the probability of them having a genetic condition. Today, it is given to all pregnant women, unless they expressly opt out. Before the roll-out of the combined test, however, women would have had an initial scan only later on, at around sixteen weeks – if they had one at all.* In other words, it's coincidence. The twelve-week scan may unwittingly reinforce older ideas about when a pregnancy feels more certain, more real, but its ubiquity in pregnancy care today may also mean that the twelve-week 'rule' is much more of an absolute decree for us than it ever was for our mothers or grandmothers.

That first visual proof of your pregnancy is an undeniably powerful moment, though. Research has shown that ultrasound increases the strength of foetal attachment in parents-to-be of both genders – and also in grandparents-to-be when they are given the opportunity to attend such scans.[6] Professor Macklon suggests to me that healthcare professionals are not immune to this seeing-is-believing effect, either, which may have unintended consequences for miscarriage care. He reflects that medics may overemphasize the significance of seeing a heartbeat, in terms of ongoing miscarriage risk, because for them, as the ones performing the scan, it's the first moment the pregnancy becomes real. The flipside of this, he says, is that it creates a hierarchy in terms of how healthcare professionals value miscarriages, devaluing losses that occur before a scan can be done. 'One of the reasons we assume women should handle a

---

* My mum tells me she did not have any ultrasound scans at all in her pregnancies with me or my brother in the 1980s, or when she had my sister, who was born just before the start of the new millennium.

"biochemical" pregnancy better than, say, a miscarriage after an early scan, is because of the importance that professionals place on saying, "Look, I can see a foetal heart,"' he says. 'When that then gets lost, it's no longer just an affair for the couple; other people have given it a certain value, which in a biochemical pregnancy hasn't happened yet.'

This all goes some way to explain why the twelve-week rule – which for some mutates into a belief that it's somehow 'bad luck' to announce a pregnancy any earlier – has persisted where other superstitions born out of historic fears around childbirth, such as not bringing a pram into the house before a baby is born, have all but faded away. Yet what about the growing number of women who now get this 'first look' at their pregnancy even earlier than twelve weeks, thanks to the rising popularity and affordability of early private scans, often marketed to women as a fun, bonding experience rather than a diagnostic service? Add to that the prevalence of IVF treatment, which involves bearing witness to a pregnancy right from the moment a fertilized egg is transferred back into the uterus. Given the apparent power of visual proof, why haven't the norms around announcing a pregnancy started to shift earlier, too? What else might dictate why someone would want to wait to announce a pregnancy long after they are convinced of its reality?

The missing factor here is the tension that exists in an experience that is 'private and public at the same time', as Dr Kilshaw puts it. Pregnancy is an intimate thing and therefore who we tell is no small judgement. Yet, we are not, as a rule, governed by the prudish attitudes surrounding women's bodies and sex that dominated in the past. We no longer feel we have to hide away coyly for the duration of a pregnancy, as previous generations did. We don't, on the whole, stigmatize pregnancy if someone isn't married. The semi-naked bump-shot is all but inevitable for a certain kind of celebrity today. In short, there's less shame attached to pregnancy than has ever existed in history. It must be the threat of miscarriage, then, that prevents us from being as open about early pregnancy as we are about the later weeks. And, while we might assume otherwise, there are reasons that disclosing a miscarriage might be even harder in our current climate. Far from existing linearly, and only recently starting to fade, there is perhaps *more* secrecy and shame around miscarriage today than in the past.

When the historian Shannon Withycombe set out to write a history of miscarriage in the nineteenth century, based on women's own accounts of their experience, she 'initially assumed that miscarriage would be considered a failure or a shameful event' – that the feelings many recount about pregnancy loss today would be echoed back to us, amplified by the importance that society placed on motherhood back then. 'I rushed into the archives, thumbing through yellowed diaries and flaking letters from 150 years ago, certain I would find descriptions of grief, frustration, depression, or shame,' she recalls. 'Or maybe I would find nothing at all. Perhaps women of the 19th century kept quiet on the issues of miscarriage, feeling ashamed of their failures, or unable to discuss such a private, embarrassing topic.'[7] Instead, what she uncovered was that while, yes, some women experienced miscarriage with sadness, many others described the relief, thankfulness, even joy they felt afterwards. At first, Withycombe couldn't make sense of these reactions, until she started to put them into the full context of what these women's lives were like. For some, a miscarriage would otherwise have been their tenth child in as many years. For others, they discovered they were pregnant (again) in the shadow of an army's advance. These women's attitudes to miscarriage were, she saw, completely understandable in light of the economic and social realities they lived with. What's more, for them the (misplaced) shame of losing a pregnancy didn't exist in the way it does for many women today because, thanks to medical and cultural ambiguities around life inside the womb, it wasn't seen as a failure of motherhood.

Only a very unimaginative minority today see motherhood as being a woman's primary and exclusive duty. It's presumed that most women will work outside the home, alongside raising families, if they choose to have them. And yet miscarriage is more closely aligned now with a sense of deep, personal failure than it seems to have been when the main social role allocated to women was mothering, at a time when we couldn't vote, own property, live or travel alone. Why? Where is the shame coming from? What could it be about our own economic and social realities that makes it so hard to disclose an early pregnancy – or its loss? Could it be coming from the modern workplace? Put it this way: I don't think it's a coincidence that the twelve-week rule endures while the working world is still such an unforgiving place to be a mother.

Women's employment rates fall sharply after having children, from around 90 per cent to 75 per cent, according to a 2021 analysis by the Institute for Fiscal Studies.[8] For mothers who do stay in the workplace, there is an equally sharp reduction in the average number of hours worked – falling from around forty to less than thirty per week. However, the same is not true of men after the birth of their children. In fact, even when a woman earns more than her male partner, she is much more likely to leave her job or reduce her paid working hours than a man who earns more than his female partner. It would be wrong to characterize this as a product of women's uncomplicated choice to spend more time with their children. Almost half (46 per cent) of British employers agree it is reasonable to ask women if they have young children during the recruitment process, the Equality and Human Rights Commission found in 2018,[9] while the same research suggests an estimated 54,000 women a year are pushed out of their jobs due to pregnancy or taking maternity leave. What's more, backing up what many women already suspected, there is evidence that employers discriminate pre-emptively, being less likely to promote women they perceive might soon have children – or they just don't hire them in the first place.[10] With all this in mind, why would anyone reveal a pregnancy any sooner than they had to? And why would you risk your employer finding out about a pregnancy that didn't make it, especially if you don't yet have children?

I *did* tell work about my first miscarriage, but that isn't to say I didn't feel anxious about doing so. I worried even as I was typing out the email to my editor that it was the wrong decision. Your legal position after a miscarriage feels precarious. What I know now, but didn't then, is that any time off requested or required for pregnancy loss before twenty-four weeks should be recorded by your employer as pregnancy-related sickness, which means that it then cannot be used against you in disciplinary proceedings or if they start making redundancies. There is also no time limit to the amount of pregnancy-related sickness leave you can take, although your GP may need to sign it off.[11] New laws that mandate statutory paid leave after a miscarriage, like the one introduced by the New Zealand government in 2021, have been applauded for their part in breaking down the taboo around pregnancy loss. Yet while policies like this undeniably help validate the impact miscarriage can have as a kind of bereavement, and are better than nothing at all, they also still assume that women will feel able to *ask* for this kind of leave in the first place.

And our reluctance at letting employers know about our miscarriages may run deeper than blunt practicalities or statistic-backed anxieties about career progression. The sense of failure so many describe after pregnancy loss speaks to the existence of some other, more essential fear: that to reveal a miscarriage also reveals something about ourselves that we would rather remain hidden. Shortly after my first miscarriage,

I was asked to move departments at work. Rationally, I don't think the two events were linked. I didn't lose out financially – in fact, I was given a pay rise. And yet, I still feared it was a demotion in all but name. I felt ashamed that I had somehow allowed the reproductive chaos of my personal life to leach into my working life.

We are sold on the importance and virtue of being in control; of deciding when and how – especially when it comes to fertility.[12] 'It's been made a kind of neo-liberal responsibility,' suggests Dr Kilshaw, for women in the UK and similar Anglo-European societies. And miscarriage, of course, disrupts all of that. It's unpredictable and messy, both emotionally and physically. We can't control it, which perhaps we internalize as a failure of self-control. Add to this a background awareness of what the sociologist Shelley J. Correll has called a 'cultural bias against mothers' – unlike fathers, working women who have children are perceived as less reliable and less capable – and the negative spiral leads inexorably to shame. Because, after a miscarriage, this kind of cultural bias hits you twice, once on the way up, once on the way down: you fear the kind of failure that attaches itself to all mothers in the workplace, and you have also failed to become a mother. The insinuation is that you are doubly unreliable, doubly incapable.

Now that I am self-employed, I no longer have a boss's expectations to manage with this fifth pregnancy.* But the irony is that, as much as I think the custom of waiting until twelve weeks does a lot to keep miscarriage hidden, my own

---

* Freedom from the traditional workplace could be a reason there seems to be a gulf between the number of celebrities and social media influencers talking about miscarriage and the lived reality of a lot of women, who still don't feel able to share in the same way. It would explain why we have a conflicted sense of whether it really is a taboo: why it still feels invisible, even as high-profile people are talking about it.

miscarriages have made it all the harder to share pregnancy news.

At the hospital, I squeak my name to the receptionist. We are early. This may be our twelve-week scan, but it has taken us a total of forty-eight weeks of pregnancy to get here. And now that we are, I'm really not sure if I can wait another twenty minutes. Fortunately, they see us almost straight away. I have my spiel prepared for the sonographer.

'A bit anxious . . . four miscarriages,' I say, handing over my fat sheaf of notes.

'Thank you for telling me,' she says, as I lie down on the scanning couch. There is the briefest of pauses. Unlike in previous scans, I don't have time to mentally rehearse the ways she might diagnose another disappointment.

'OK, here's your baby.'

Whereas in previous pregnancies there has only been cavernous blackness on the ultrasound monitor at this stage, now it is filled with wobbling movement: the grey outline of a head and a tiny, round tummy – a waving, wondrous sea creature emerging from the dark.

'They're a wriggler,' the sonographer tells us, smiling. She adjusts the transducer, reasserting its pressure against my abdomen. I grip Dan's hand and we watch as the baby somersaults for us. I am almost afraid to look away in case they stop; in case I miss any of it. I want every second of this moment, this life. I could sit here all day watching them. Our baby. The only one who has made it this far.

7

'Products of conception'

(January 2020 – 13 weeks pregnant)

On New Year's Day, I throw up. Just once. Crouched on the bathroom floor, still in my pyjamas, I can hear Dan and our friends down in the living room, laughing as they try to play a board game their children got for Christmas: the morning after the night before. Last night, we'd had dinner and then huddled together in our garden to watch the fireworks across the valley, laughing and cheering as the rockets erupted and fell to earth. It's pleasingly ironic to me that I am the one feeling worse for wear this morning, when I had been the first to go to bed, sober. This is now the most pregnant I have ever been. Everything from here is untrodden ground. This, coupled with the fresh memory of the ultrasound from yesterday, means I can relax into something approaching enjoyment. On a whim after the scan, I bought a new pair of thick, generously sized leggings – not official maternity wear, as it still feels too soon for that, but a concession to this pregnancy all the same. When I pull them on, I feel a prickle of optimism, as though it has jumped from the fabric, charging my skin like static. Later, when we head out for an afternoon walk, we take a group picture. Only my face is visible and, anyway, there is no outward sign of my condition yet, at least not under coats and scarfs. But it occurs to me all the same that it is the first picture I have of myself in this pregnancy. For the first time in more than two months, I start to feel expansive and hopeful.

It doesn't last, of course. As we get further away from the last scan, the optimism leaks out of me like air from a pinhole puncture. The hospital has agreed to give us an extra scan, at eighteen weeks, for reassurance, but that is still over a month away. And while I know the risk of pregnancy loss is significantly lower now, miscarriages after the first trimester do still happen. It's estimated that 1–2 per cent of pregnancies end in miscarriage beyond thirteen weeks, although I cannot find an exact number for how many late miscarriages happen each year in the UK – once again, we don't include them in the official maternity statistics. This is despite the fact that a late miscarriage, which is defined as any pregnancy that ends before twenty-four weeks, may be much closer in kind to the experience of having an extremely pre-term birth or a stillborn baby. Waters can break, dramatically, noticeably. It can come with painful, prolonged contractions. If a late miscarriage is diagnosed at a scan, labour may have to be induced. The notion that twelve weeks represents a 'safe point', reinforced by traditions and trends around pregnancy announcements, further heightens the taboo around these later miscarriages. If few pregnancy books acknowledge the possibility of early miscarriage in any real depth, even fewer broach the prospect of losing a baby later on. Unlike early pregnancy loss, which is treated as an unremarkable reproductive hiccup, barely worthy of deep consideration, late miscarriage is hidden away as too rare and too distressing even to mention. It's a harsh no man's land that we've created. The expectation is set up that babies will not die after this stage and yet there is still relatively little doctors can do to intervene if a pregnancy is threatened before the threshold of viability. Sometimes, if the cervix is found to be opening after sixteen weeks, an emergency procedure can be performed known as a rescue stitch – but this is not possible if you are already bleeding or having contractions. Likewise, for babies born before twenty-two weeks, it is vanishingly rare for doctors to attempt resuscitation; indeed, it is not recommended in the UK. For babies born in the 'pre-viable' hinterland, approaching twenty-four weeks, medical decisions are complex and require enormous sensitivity and expertise. And if a baby dies in utero before twenty-four weeks, no legal record is kept: no birth certificate, no death certificate. Some women also find themselves in a grey area in terms of their medical care – they are beyond the remit of early-pregnancy units, but a busy labour ward may not be where they want to be, either, especially if the miscarriage seems inevitable. What's more, women report being turned away from maternity services. An NHS England report from 2013 suggested that many wards have rules about the point in pregnancy at which they will admit women – the cut-off varied between maternity units, but most commonly was twenty weeks.[1] Any earlier in pregnancy and women would be directed to general gynaecology instead. 'To my ears, all I heard was that my baby was not worthy of midwifery care as it wasn't big enough,' recounts Ali Stewart, a midwife, who was turned away from the nearest maternity unit when her waters broke at sixteen weeks, in 2017. A few days later, her daughter Elodie was born silent – at a different hospital, which allowed Ali to use a delivery suite, like any other labouring mother. Elodie weighed just 100g but had 'perfect tiny feet and tiny toes', says Ali. As is common with babies lost at this stage, Elodie was so small it was another few days after her birth before her parents could be told her sex, something that was only discernible through genetic testing.

The potential known causes of late miscarriages are broadly similar to the possible known reasons for recurrent miscarriage and women tend to be offered the same investigations for either kind of loss. However, unlike early miscarriage, late miscarriage is considered to be a rare enough event that it should always warrant medical follow-up. The fact that, medically, late miscarriages are considered rare is of little comfort to me now, though. After all, 1 per cent – or one in 100 cases – is roughly the same prevalence as the number of people affected by recurrent miscarriage. These days I find it hard to trust in probability. Just as I find it hard to trust in my body. I had hoped that the sudden violent sickness that had gripped me on New Year's Day would persist for a little while, an escalation of my symptoms and a kind of evidence that I could use to quiet my brain's wilder conspiracy theories. But it proves to be a one-off. The Hollywood-style, throwing-up-in-your-handbag morning sickness continues to elude me, as it has done the previous four times. I try not to think about what this might mean.

It helps that we are still camping out in the new house, sleeping on an air mattress in our bedroom, while we wait for furniture to be delivered. Our half-made state gives us plenty to do. I throw myself into decorating. I discover a new interest in buying old things, antiques and second-hand oddities – a funny green table with curving edges like the blades of a leaf; a wooden chest that smells like earth – while small tasks like buying plants and getting a new radio for the kitchen suddenly seem disproportionately important.

What I am trying to create, I realize, is noise and activity, and a sense of the new house being alive. Because what I am afraid of most is stillness. Because, without necessarily acknowledging the thought at full tilt, I am desperate to feel this baby move – though I know this is unlikely to happen for another few weeks, at least. I am no longer bleeding, which is a relief of a kind. But now, what I fear as much as sighting blood when I go to the loo is a so-called 'missed' or 'silent' miscarriage – that is, the baby will stop growing, its heart will stop beating, and my body will not notice. After all, this is how we found out we'd lost our previous two pregnancies.

Like late miscarriage, this is a nuance of how and when miscarriages happen that is largely missing from our shared understanding. Many people remain unaware of the possibility of 'missed' miscarriage right up until it happens to them. I only learned of its existence in the hours I spent online in the aftermath of my first miscarriage, haunted by the extra twist of cruelty that you could walk into a scan at twelve weeks completely unsuspecting. That too-still scan and those whispered apologies are enough of a blow when you've had a morning of blood loss to prepare for the possibility, let alone when there has been no clue.

A missed miscarriage is an experience that the anthropologist Susie Kilshaw describes as 'really shocking'. Dr Kilshaw's academic interest in reproductive loss grew out of her personal experience, her first pregnancy having ended in a missed miscarriage, discovered at her dating scan, when she should have been thirteen weeks pregnant. She, too, had no idea such a thing could happen. 'That was quite destabilizing, as an educated woman in my thirties who was prepared for pregnancy,' she tells me. 'I was similar to many women in that I'd learned a lot about conception and how *not* to get pregnant; what vitamins to take and these sorts of things. I knew about miscarriage, but I really had no understanding about how varied the experience can be, physically.'

Neither did I. I have had surgery following a missed miscarriage twice now – for pregnancies number three and number four. Both bodies were removed from my body at the same hospital. The first time, I'd gone along to join a trial looking at symptoms in the first trimester, attracted by the promise of weekly early scans. When the softly spoken research fellow had scanned me and broken the news, I was led to a private, boxed-off room, where I could wait for someone to talk to me about my 'options'. Cloistered in that small waiting room with walls painted pale peach – a shade someone must have deemed inoffensive – I sat with the improbability of what had just happened. Hadn't I less than thirty minutes ago retched at the salt tang of a stranger's aftershave on the Tube? How could that happen when the baby was dead already? How could my body get this so wrong? How could it not know?

So this is what it has come to, I thought to myself. *Not only can I not stay pregnant, my body is so confused it does not know how to miscarry, either.*

As much as a missed miscarriage can feel like a different 'type' of miscarriage – a new way in which your body does not appear to work the way it should – it does not necessarily have a different biological meaning from one that announces itself with blood and cramps. Instead, like very early miscarriage, it is another reproductive experience that has been 'created' by access to technology, specifically early ultrasound. For previous generations, it was rare for a miscarriage to be diagnosed on a scan before a woman herself had any suspicion the pregnancy had ended. Dr Hanine Fourie is a clinical research fellow in early pregnancy and ultrasound. She is also the infinitely kind, calm person who diagnosed my third miscarriage, as I attempted to join the research study to which she was recruiting [EPOS-2 (Early Pregnancy events and Outcomes Study)] at Queen Charlotte's and Chelsea Hospital, in London. 'Missed miscarriage, especially prior to twelve weeks of pregnancy, may be a clinically created entity,' she explains. 'If you scanned everybody early, you may diagnose more missed miscarriages, whereas if you scan later, the miscarriage process may have started.'

And the relative newness of missed miscarriage as an experience may explain, at least in part, why we are still unfamiliar

with the idea. Before the introduction of the combined screening test and a routine twelve-week ultrasound scan in the early
2000s, diagnosing early pregnancy loss on a scan did not really
happen. Professor Ana Nikčević is a professor of psychology
and mental health at Kingston University and practitioner
psychologist who, in the late 1990s, was asked to conduct
research into the psychological impact of bringing screening
and scanning forward to the end of the first trimester. 'At the
time, diagnosis of pregnancy loss at a scan was a new phenomenon,' she tells me. Before that, if women did have a scan at all,
it tended to be later on in pregnancy, by which point most miscarriages would already have happened. 'They were trying to
bring forward earlier screening for all pregnant women,' she
says. 'But this meant that the end of a pregnancy became something a doctor communicates.'

Unravelling exactly what's happened in a missed miscarriage
is difficult. It can be hard to judge when the pregnancy actually
ended; for how long this has evaded detection. 'It's difficult
because, for a pregnancy which is chromosomally abnormal,
the foetus won't be growing at the same rate as a normal pregnancy,' explains Dr Fourie. 'Even if you measure a foetus that
is much smaller, that's maybe three weeks earlier than someone's dates suggest, that doesn't mean that's when the miscarriage
happened.' What's more, 'You're measuring such small struc-
tures and there can be changes after the pregnancy stops
developing, so the foetus may look smaller compared to when
it stopped growing,' she adds.

Even so, Dr Fourie says, people often feel an urgent need to
know when the pregnancy ended. When she was working in
early-pregnancy assessment units, she found it was often the first
question asked. 'I sometimes wondered if people were looking
to find a reason – that they wanted to attribute it to something
that happened in their life or that they did,' she tells me.

As well as that instinct to blame ourselves, I also wonder if this impulse to know the exact time of death is because we are trying to quantify what we are allowed to feel. We are looking for a biological schema to define the parameters of our grief. On one level, we may do this because other people's responses to miscarriage have been hidden away from us and therefore we don't know what is 'normal' or proportionate. But it may also come from our deeply ingrained belief that there are hierarchies of bereavement. We cleave to this idea that some losses are worse than others and that there are appropriate levels of mourning. Yet all around us there is evidence of how grief defies neat categorization. The loss of a parent does not feel the same for everyone. For some, the death of a much-loved pet will floor them in a way the loss of an estranged human relative did not. For others, the acute stage of grief comes not with the last breath, but during the slow, unfurling illness that takes the person they love to somewhere unreachable. An aching absence can be created by the death of a colleague we saw every day yet didn't even know their address or middle name. And, I concede, not everyone will feel the way I have done about miscarriages.

It is a hard habit to shake, though, this emotional stratification. There is a little part of me that still clings to gestational age as a shorthand for significance – even though I have reassured many others to the contrary, and even though I know, at my core, I don't consider a miscarriage that happened at five or six weeks to someone else to be 'lesser' than my own, later miscarriages. I also know that when I tell the story of my first miscarriage, I like to insist a little too much how close we were to that twelve-week scan, as if that meant anything at all. As though it's not entirely possible it could have ended weeks earlier, just like the other three.

When doctors cannot reliably tell us when a pregnancy ended, many of us try to trace it for ourselves, connecting the dots with our symptoms – or lack thereof. 'There can be subtle signs,' says Hanine Fourie. 'Like loss of breast tenderness. That's a hormonal symptom of the progesterone: often when women lose that symptom it can be a sign of progesterone dropping.' Then there's nausea. Despite the millions it affects each year, it's not known exactly what causes morning sickness, but one factor is believed to be the pregnancy hormone HCG. What *is* known is that nausea in pregnancy is often a positive sign. 'It's a very reassuring symptom – there have been good studies to show that if women have nausea and vomiting, their risk of miscarriage is low,' says Dr Fourie. Research using a validated, clinical scale known as the 'PUQE' score (yes, really)* to measure the extent of morning sickness has also suggested that the risk relates to the severity of someone's nausea, too. 'If you have a high "PUQE" score, you have a lower risk of miscarriage than someone with a lower score,' adds Dr Fourie.[†]

However, while some women do report feeling less sick just before they learn they have miscarried, an absence or change in nausea is not always a cause for concern. 'HCG peaks at ten weeks and then it does naturally go down, so many – but not all – women will have a very normal experience where their nausea and vomiting gets better from ten weeks,' says Dr Fourie. There is also some evidence that morning sickness is at least in part genetic, whether that's a tendency to extreme nausea or lack of nausea.[2]

---

* PUQE stands for Pregnancy-Unique Quantification of Emesis and Nausea, a dubious acronym that feels a lot less like a harmless joke to an anxiously pregnant woman or, I would imagine, to someone suffering from the extreme and debilitating morning-sickness condition hyperemesis gravidarum.
[†] Even hyperemesis gravidarum does not seem to confer a higher risk of miscarriage, although it can raise the likelihood of a premature birth, as well as a baby being small for their gestational age. What's more, the condition can be so unbearable, an estimated one in seven women feel they have no choice but to terminate their pregnancy.

In a pregnancy after a previous miscarriage, and especially after one diagnosed on a scan, the thought of missing some clue from inside your own body can be all-consuming. This intense anxiety about symptoms is something that healthcare professionals don't always fully appreciate, says Dr Sarah Bailey, who is the lead nurse for recurrent-miscarriage care at University Hospital Southampton NHS Foundation Trust. 'I don't think they understand the hypervigilance,' she tells me. 'When someone rings and says "I've got a bit of tummy pain" or "My breasts don't hurt any more", it's so easy for healthcare professionals to brush this away.' While she tries to reassure her own patients that symptoms can vary day-to-day, she notes that fears about their absence are mainstays of discussion on online support groups. 'It just makes me think we're not getting it right, because there's a whole community out there feeling desperate,' she says.

At fifteen weeks, my pregnancy symptoms vanish overnight. I'd been expecting to slowly feel better – less sick, less tired – now that I was in the second trimester, but this is as if a switch has been tripped. It's like waking up the day after a hangover and remembering, with elation, what your body feels like unpoisoned. My face is less grey. My limbs no longer feel heavy. And I feel like drinking a coffee, for the first time in months. I am pleased and then completely panicked. I remind myself that this could well just be the second-trimester uplift that everyone promises. More grimly, I remind myself that just as I've had symptoms tail off in pregnancies I've miscarried weeks later, I've also had miscarriages in spite of symptoms that remained strong.

Rather than simply expecting women and pregnant people to accept the unknowability of vague, fluctuating symptoms, some researchers are now attempting to find objective biomarkers that could mean a miscarriage could one day be diagnosed – or ruled out – from blood tests.[3] For example, there is some evidence that a protein called AFP (alpha-fetoprotein), which is made by the yolk sac in early pregnancy, is shed into the maternal bloodstream in higher amounts in pregnancies that are struggling or haven't implanted properly. 'But these markers are not yet robust enough or sensitive enough to be used in large groups of women,' says Hanine Fourie.

Dr Fourie also points out that discoveries in this area could present new ethical dilemmas. Quite apart from the extra anxiety blood tests for miscarriage could cause, if you spot that a pregnancy is not going to continue, but at the moment is viable, what do you do?

Even if scientists do discover a way of reliably identifying more potential miscarriages at an earlier stage, and from blood tests alone, the fact that more miscarriages could then take on this 'missed' or 'silent' form is not uncomplicated or even straightforwardly preferable. Because when you have a 'missed' miscarriage, you are required to make a decision, even if what you decide is to do nothing. Just as you are getting over the shock of the diagnosis – a diagnosis you may not have known was possible until several seconds ago – you have to choose what to do next. You have to choose how to 'manage' the missed miscarriage.

If you are lucky, someone like Dr Fourie, with a voice threaded with warmth and patience, will take their time to reassure you and talk you through the choices: pills, surgery, or waiting it out. They will explain that surgical management can be a discrete, finite way of handling it. That it is the best way to get a sample if you want – and are eligible for – genetic testing of the pregnancy tissue. They will also tell you that while the more conservative option of waiting for the miscarriage to start of its own accord can be drawn-out and painful, some find in seeing the proof and process of the miscarriage for themselves something like catharsis. They will make you aware that while taking the requisite medication to bring it on is safe and effective, it doesn't always work and surgery may be required after all.* If you're really lucky, your medical team will assure you that whichever method you choose, research shows it doesn't affect your chance of conceiving again. They might also reassure you that by choosing to take medication or have surgery, you do not risk ending a pregnancy that might have been OK after all. 'We've got very safe diagnostic criteria now to diagnose miscarriage,' as Dr Fourie puts it.

But even with the best intentions and counselling, nothing will make what you pick feel like a good decision. Nothing will feel even a bit like consolation. It won't feel right. How could it? You are being forced to pick from options that are the exact opposite of what you want. Of course, you also know that you cannot stay as you are. The thought of continuing to harbour winter inside, where once there was spring, is as untenable as the thought of letting it go.

When we talk about miscarriage being a taboo, we should consider what is missing from the stories we do hear. Narratives around miscarriage are, Dr Susie Kilshaw says, 'very sanitized'. It's details like the extent of the blood loss, the type of surgery,

---

* It's been proposed that the chance of this kind of 'medical management' not working could be reduced with a different combination of medications, giving women the anti-progesterone drug mifepristone as well as the current standard drug, misoprostol. A randomized controlled trial in 2020 found this combined treatment worked 83 per cent of the time, compared to 76 per cent with the current prescription. (J. J. Chu et al., 'Mifepristone and misoprostol versus misoprostol alone for the management of missed miscarriage (MifeMiso): a randomised, double-blind, placebo-controlled trial', *Lancet*, 396:10253 (2020) 770–78: https://pubmed.ncbi.nlm.nih.gov/32853559.) This method was also found to be more cost-effective than misoprostol alone, in subsequent research. (T. E. Roberts et al., 'Cost-effectiveness of mifepristone and misoprostol versus misoprostol alone for the management of missed miscarriage: an economic evaluation based on the MifeMiso trial', *British Journal of Obstetrics and Gynaecology*, 128:9 (2021) 1534–45: https://obgyn.onlinelibrary.wiley.com/doi/10.1111/1471-0528.16737.)

or how you choose what to do when a miscarriage won't start by itself, that tend to get left out. As is the postscript to any miscarriage: that you have to decide what to do with the body (which, in an attempt at neutrality, medics tend to refer to as the 'products of conception').

This, says Dr Kilshaw, ranks high in the list of 'elements we feel very squeamish about'. Even if you opt for surgery, in which case the miscarriage will remain out of sight, if not out of mind, you have to declare what you want to do with the tissue – the body, the baby – afterwards. This is a relatively recent development. In the UK, it was only in 2015 that formal, comprehensive guidance to hospitals was issued by the Human Tissue Authority; before then, it was not uncommon for pregnancy remains – to use the coldly clinical term – to be treated as any other clinical waste. Now, national policy is that you should be told that you have options and that your personal preference and consent is paramount. This includes being offered various forms of burial and cremation. You are also entitled to have the tissue returned to you, should you wish. Equally, if you prefer not to think or talk about any of it, doctors should respect this.

Both times, after my missed miscarriages, I have declined to see, take home, or otherwise ceremonialize the bodily matter of my pregnancies. Instead, I signed my name so that, after genetic tests, the tissue could be used for medical research or else disposed of by the hospital as it saw fit. I felt no affinity with the physical residue. That was not where the meaning of this loss lived for me. I didn't miss the literal body. But still, I feel guilty about this decision. Just as I feel guilty that the fate of my two other miscarried pregnancies was to be flushed away. I find it relatively easy, now, to talk about my miscarriages. But not this. This, above everything else, still feels shameful and proscribed.

Dr Kilshaw, whose latest research is focusing on the materiality of pregnancy loss and what we do with those remains, reflects that whatever women choose or whatever happens, they often feel uneasy about it. 'It's another opportunity to worry that you've done something you shouldn't,' she tells me. 'There's no right or wrong, but we're so quick to think "Did I do the wrong thing?"' For me, it's a kind of doubt that's surely amplified by silence and not knowing what other people do. My own feelings of guilt certainly intensified when, much further down the line, I learned of other women who scattered the ashes from their miscarriage somewhere beautiful, or who buried tiny bodies in their gardens, planting something that would come into flower around what would have been their due date. Then again, I know that women who are open about these kinds of memorials are sometimes met with discomfort and disapproval from others. There is no social consensus as to what the appropriate maternal response to this kind of loss should be. Not that there should necessarily be a single sanctioned response, but in a vacuum everything feels wrong. In this ambiguous zone of pre-birth, you are made to feel as if you are not acting as enough of a mother – or that you are being too much of one.

Now, as the days crawl along to sixteen weeks, I think I feel increasingly attached to the reality of the body inside mine, as well as the 'child in mind'. I don't know when that started to shift, exactly, but I am more aware of its weight inside me. There is still no movement that I can feel. But one weekday morning, I try on a new, roomy dress and notice, for the first time, that my reflection is giving away the news I have yet to make public. As I pivot left and right in front of the bedroom mirror, it seems implausible that I could have missed the fact of my stomach until now. It is so insistently round, all of a sudden. I suppose I have been concealing myself from myself in jumpers and leggings. Still wondering if I am imagining things,

I send a badly lit selfie to one of our few friends who know. I have a bobble hat on over unwashed hair and the face I've captured is wan and expressionless, my gaze off-kilter, not looking straight at the lens.

'This is just the best sight ever,' she pings back straight away. 'Definitely pregnant.'

8

'It can't be helped'

(February 2020 – 16 weeks pregnant)

'There's no real benefit to taking it for any longer, as far as we know,' the doctor is telling me. I nod along, while silently shredding my cuticles, as I always do when I am worried. Did he have to add the 'as far as we know'?

We're at the hospital again for a routine appointment. So far, a midwife has cuffed me for my blood pressure and extracted yet more phials of blood. We are getting used to the routine now. You place one form in an in-tray of a particular colour as you enter. Your maternity notes go in another. Then there's a different form to be handed back to the receptionist on the way out. The main waiting room is lined with plastic chairs in a spectrum of primary-school colours. Dan and I are meeting with a consultant – a different face from last time – and he is saying what I knew was coming. It's time to stop taking the progesterone supplements I've been on for nearly ten weeks, the progesterone I sometimes convince myself is the only reason I'm still pregnant.

Stopping feels like severing a cord and I am afraid of what I perceive as inevitable free fall.

But I don't know how to say this. The doctor has moved on to telling me that I should probably also start taking low-dose aspirin from hereon in. Apparently, this is standard advice to reduce the risk of pre-eclampsia and growth restriction later in pregnancy. However, I have a dim recollection of being told by a consultant at the miscarriage clinic that aspirin is *not* recommended for people with a history like mine. Despite its popularity as a home remedy among women trying to conceive, I was told it can actually interfere with implantation. But perhaps I am misremembering. I feel myself frown. I progress to picking at the soft crescent of flesh behind my thumbnail. I ask whether I can just stop the progesterone overnight, or whether I should reduce the daily dose incrementally. The consultant doesn't know – though he suggests there'd be no harm in finishing up what's left of my prescription, if I wish. I say I want to speak to the clinic first before I agree to the aspirin. The consultant doesn't demur.

It makes me feel like an arse, doubting my doctors like this. After all, I did not go to medical school. I don't even have science A-levels. But there comes a point when it is hard to trust that the doctor in front of you is as read-up on the subject as you are. After all, I am only on the progesterone in the first place because I asked for it. And I want to do the right thing, the thing that gives me the best chance of bringing home this baby, far more than I want to be a compliant patient.

By my count, during our time under the recurrent-miscarriage clinic and now in this pregnancy, I have seen eight different doctors, each for barely longer than ten minutes. Almost all have been sympathetic, if briskly efficient. I do not think I would necessarily recognize any of them were we to pass each other in the supermarket, or should we happen to be waiting for the same bus. This absence of a meaningful clinical relationship is a strange environment in which to navigate so many medical unknowns – and at such a vulnerable, labile juncture in your life.

When it comes to the treatment of recurrent miscarriage, 'clinical practice is inconsistent and poorly organised' concluded the authors of a paper published in the *Lancet* in 2021.[1] The tests and subsequent therapies you may be offered vary widely across the country, even between specialist clinics. Often, even when your care is based on the most up-to-date evidence available, the only suggestion doctors can make is to try again. For people with unexplained miscarriages – like me and Dan – there is no consensus that any treatment will help.

The most fundamental hurdle is perhaps the prevailing sense of nihilism. 'There is a sense of hopelessness; that there's nothing that can be done,' says Arri Coomarasamy, a professor of gynaecology and reproductive medicine, and the director of the UK's National Centre for Miscarriage Research. 'So that impedes progress.'

Then there is the inescapable truth that miscarriage predominantly happens to women's bodies, with all the historical and medical baggage that bequeaths. It's quite the inheritance. There is a long tradition of ignoring, minimizing, or even denying what women report about their own physical health, coupled with a lack of interest in giving women access to detailed, accurate information about their bodies. It was, remember, 1971 before a woman could even find out for herself without a doctor's approval if she was pregnant (and, often, they didn't approve). The first medics working to develop ultrasound scanning techniques for pregnancy were actually laughed at by hospital colleagues, who apparently couldn't see the merit in such a project.[2] Dr Marlena Fejzo was also met with laughter when she announced that she wanted to conduct a study into the genetics of the extreme morning-sickness condition hyperemesis gravidarum in the late 1990s. Our health is still taken less seriously. Our pain goes underestimated and under-medicated.[3] We are less likely to be referred for certain kinds of surgery.[4] Conditions where women make up the majority of patients, such as CFS/ME or fibromyalgia, receive disproportionately less research funding.[5] Conditions affecting the female reproductive system, such as endometriosis, fare particularly badly, despite their prevalence – attracting less than 2.1 per cent of total research spending in the UK (and that figure also includes childbirth-related conditions).[6] Meanwhile, in 2021, 41 per cent of UK universities did not have mandatory menopause education on the curriculum for medical students. What's more, 'the practice of medicine was built using research that was done primarily on male cells, male animals, and male test subjects', notes the geneticist and researcher Dr Sharon Moalem in his book *The Better Half*.[7] The US's National Institutes of Health didn't legally require clinical trials to include women as well as men until 1993. Despite evidence that male and female cells behave differently, early-stage or 'pre-clinical' research has frequently relied on male cells alone. As the writer and feminist campaigner Caroline Criado Perez puts it brilliantly in her book *Invisible Women*, 'How many treatments have women missed out on because they had no effect on the male cells on which they were exclusively tested?'

Adding to this legacy is the fact that, for most of human history, pregnancy has not been considered a medical matter anyway (despite the vast numbers of women who have died in childbirth or following miscarriages). Even in the modern medical era, 'obstetrics and gynaecology used to be a bit of a Cinderella specialty; it didn't get as much funding as other things, such as liver disease or gut disease', says Professor Phillip Bennett, director of the Institute of Reproductive and Developmental Biology at Imperial College London. While things are improving, he says, pregnancy research, as a whole, remains underfunded – let alone miscarriage specifically. A review published in 2020 found that for every £1 spent on pregnancy care in the NHS, less than 1p is spent on pregnancy research. This, the researchers concluded, was far less generous than in other areas of health.[8]

Pregnancy is also difficult for scientists to study in real time, acknowledges Professor Nick Macklon, of the London Women's Clinic. 'By its nature, studying it might disrupt it,' he says. Meanwhile, animal models are often unsuitable because, when it comes to reproduction, humans seem to be a species apart.

There have, of course, been huge strides in some areas of reproductive science – but miscarriage is not one of them. How is it we have worked out how to intervene in order to start a life in a lab – via IVF – but not how to help sustain it in the earliest weeks inside the body?*

There are prosaic explanations for why the treatment of miscarriage remains chaotic and, more often than not, a source of despair. Miscarriage – or even pregnancy loss more broadly – is not a subspecialty in medicine that doctors can train in. 'You can specialize in IVF and infertility, foetal and maternal medicine, laparoscopic surgery, or cancer, but there is no specific specialty in miscarriage,' says Professor Hassan Shehata, a consultant obstetrician and gynaecologist who runs the UK's Centre for Reproductive Immunology and Pregnancy in Surrey. It's a similar picture in the US – subspecialties for ob-gyn include female pelvic medicine and reconstructive surgery, infertility, and complex family planning, covering contraception and abortion, but not pregnancy loss. Accordingly, Professor Shehata describes miscarriage care as 'a mixed bag'. 'Couples can be referred to a specific

* Indeed, for all that IVF is now an intensively researched, rigorously controlled, highly medicated process, with different drug regimens or 'protocols' that can be personalized and tweaked to optimize the number of eggs a woman produces, if your embryos repeatedly do not implant or you miscarry later on, fertility clinics often have few answers other than 'try again'.

miscarriage service, but they can also end up seeing a gynaecologist or sent to a fertility clinic. So, the experience and how you manage future pregnancies will be very different,' he tells me.

Currently, in the UK, it can take months to be referred to a recurrent-miscarriage clinic. And that's if there is a specialist service available in your area in the first place. In Wales, for example, there are no specialist recurrent-miscarriage clinics at all; instead you are referred to a local gynaecologist, who may or may not have much experience in miscarriage. What's more, as a campaign led by Jessica Evans and Fair Treatment for the Women of Wales has highlighted, despite the lack of home-grown services, recurrent-miscarriage patients also face protracted battles to be referred to specialist services across the border in England.

For obstetrician and miscarriage specialist Professor Siobhan Quenby, it's not so much that there aren't any treatment options for recurrent-miscarriage patients; it's the will to try them that's lacking. 'There are tons of things we can try now,' she tells me. Professor Quenby is a remarkably ebullient woman. When you hear her speak about miscarriage, you cannot help but feel a rare spark of optimism. I have seen her give rousing research presentations, shod in cheerful, floral-print brogues. She radiates the unmistakeable energy of someone who can get things done. Professor Quenby is director of the Biomedical Research Unit in Reproductive Health based at University Hospital, Coventry. The unit is trying to better understand how the lining of the womb behaves and contributes to miscarriage. People who have had at least one miscarriage or IVF implantation failure can ask to be referred here by their GP for various tests, including having a biopsy taken from the lining of their womb.

Research and treatment here often contributes to ongoing studies. For example, in 2020 Professor Quenby and colleagues published a study that showed how a repurposed diabetes drug,

sitagliptin, seemed to reduce the risk of miscarriage by boost-
ing the number of stem cells in the womb lining.[9] These cells
are responsible for renewing the lining and for reducing inflammation, making the womb lining more pregnancy-'friendly'.
Sitagliptin increased stem-cell counts by an average of 68 per
cent and, more importantly, in the twelve months following
treatment, 'none of the women lost genetically normal pregnancies', explains Professor Quenby. For people who repeatedly
miscarry 'normal' embryos, 'the problem will most likely be in
the lining of the womb', she believes. Specifically, some women
who have recurrent miscarriage seem to have an imbalance of
types of cell in the uterus lining, with fewer of the helpful stem
cells and more of what are known as senescent cells, that is
aged, 'stressed out' cells, which don't or cannot support a pregnancy in the same way. 'It's still only a small pilot trial, but it is
fantastically exciting,' she says of the results. 'It's the first time
in a long time that there's been a potential new drug treatment
for miscarriage.'

Previously, the unit has also looked at whether the steroid
prednisolone can help reduce miscarriage risk by lowering the
number of a type of immune cell in the uterus called NK or
'natural killer' cells. And an ongoing trial, led by Professor
Quenby, is now looking at whether the antibiotic doxycycline
can reduce chronic inflammation of the womb lining known as
endometritis (which some women may not know they have)
and whether that in turn can reduce their risk of miscarriage.
Professor Quenby also frequently prescribes progesterone for
her patients, while in some particular cases she might offer metformin (a drug which lowers blood sugar and insulin levels and
has also been found to reduce the risk of pregnancy loss in
people who have polycystic ovary syndrome) and/or blood-
thinning medication.[10]

Something all these potential treatments have in common –
you might have noticed – is that they are all existing, well-known

medications that are being repurposed. This, Professor Shehata suggests to me, is another reason that progress in treating and preventing miscarriage has lagged behind, even as we've made enormous leaps in other areas of fertility medicine. Unlike, say, IVF-drug protocols or egg-freezing, with miscarriage medicine 'there's no pharmaceutical company back-up', he says. There just doesn't seem to be the same financial incentive to develop or study new therapies that might help people stay pregnant.

And while an expert in recurrent pregnancy loss such as Professor Quenby may legitimately feel she has a range of options to offer her patients, depending on their particular history, there is a big stumbling block when it comes to wider practice. 'There is no high-quality evidence for *any* treatment to prevent miscarriages,' or so an analysis published in the *Lancet* in 2021 concluded (of which Professor Quenby is one of the co-authors).[11] This doesn't mean treatments such as progesterone, anti-coagulant medication, metformin, or levothyroxine (a synthetic thyroid hormone), which were all considered by the *Lancet* analysis, definitely don't help or that there's no basis for offering them – but without the best-quality evidence, there may be reluctance to try. Certainly, the NHS is unlikely to recommend any treatment that doesn't satisfy the highest standards of proof.

However, obtaining this sort of evidence for miscarriage treatments is not straightforward. Even if funding is secured – and we've seen how this is an underfunded area – it can be difficult recruiting women to trials for prospective treatments. For a long time, the 'gold standard' in medical research has been randomized controlled trials, which means that patients are allocated at random either the actual treatment or a placebo. Ideally, not only will the patients not know if they're getting the real deal, but the trial doctors won't either (known as a 'double-blind' study). The trouble is, as Professor Shehata tells me, 'women feel they don't have time to take part in a study – they want the actual treatment'. There's a frustrating kind of irony here and it's a conflict I understand deeply. On the one hand, you desperately wish there was better evidence and greater clarity. On the other, you do not feel that you, personally, can help create such evidence and clarity. You fear running out the clock on your fertile years. You also fear reaching the end of your stamina: your hope muscles will, surely, hit the wall at some point. Either way, you feel on borrowed time. It's a problem that's exacerbated by the fact that many of the treatments still being studied may be relatively easy to get from a private fertility doctor (if you can afford it). When I asked my NHS clinic if they'd prescribe the progesterone, it was while knowing full well that if they said no, I would try to obtain a prescription privately. If I'd been offered a 50:50 chance of getting the treatment or a placebo as part of a trial, would I have felt able to agree to such a gamble? I can't say for certain I would. And I'm clearly not alone. One researcher tells me that at their hospital, which has a large miscarriage clinic and was trying to conduct a placebo-controlled trial, they recruited one suitable patient over the course of a whole year.

Even when major, high-quality studies *are* conducted into preventative therapies for miscarriage, the results have a history of being disappointingly inconclusive. Take the progesterone that I am currently on. The 2019 PRISM trial, which I have used as the basis for persuading my doctors to let me try it, is far from the first study into the hormone's possible benefits. Indeed, disputes have raged among medics and researchers as to its effectiveness pretty much since its inception. A synthetic form of the hormone was first developed in 1934 and it began to be used by doctors and trialled as a way of preventing miscarriages not long after, in the 1940s. The rationale behind this was that scientists knew from – rather barbaric-sounding – animal studies that progesterone is absolutely vital for pregnancy. When the structure that produces progesterone in early pregnancy, the corpus luteum, was removed, animals inevitably miscarried. Therefore the thinking was that extra progesterone could help to support pregnancy, perhaps because women who miscarried had lower-than-normal levels of the hormone. However, researchers were throwing cold water over this idea as early as 1953. A controlled trial published in the *British Medical Journal* that year, which compared the live-birth rates in 113 women who'd had two or more previous miscarriages, concluded that it made no significant difference, as the control group seemed to do just as well as those given progesterone. This was a starkly different finding to the work of previous doctors, the study authors noted.[12]

Within my own lifespan as a recurrent-miscarriage patient, the evidence pendulum has swung back and forth and back again. Progesterone seemed to be firmly off the treatment agenda after my first three miscarriages. This was due to recently published results from what was, at the time, the largest-ever study into progesterone for miscarriage, but which found no significant benefit of giving it to women with a history of recurrent loss.[13] However, in 2018, a few months after my fourth miscarriage, a review of the available evidence by the respected Cochrane group, which pooled the results of thirteen smaller trials, concluded that, in fact, for women with unexplained recurrent miscarriage, supplementary progesterone *might* reduce miscarriage rates in subsequent pregnancies.[14] Then, less than a year later, came the PRISM trial – the trial I used to make the case to my doctors for progesterone this time around – and things shifted a little more in progesterone's favour.

But why, after more than half a century of clinical research, is it still so hard to say whether progesterone might help – or, indeed, any treatment for recurrent miscarriage? Perhaps it would become clearer if we knew exactly what progesterone is supposed to do in the body to prevent miscarriage in the first place. Because, at the moment, we don't know. We know it's vital for pregnancy. But we don't know exactly how or why.

'That sort of work still needs to happen,' Professor Coomar-asamy tells me. 'In a way, we've created the evidence; now we need to go and explain why this may be the case.' Professor Macklon, for one, believes that until we do more of what he calls 'basic science to understand the mechanisms of early loss' we will struggle to produce convincing evidence for miscar-riage treatments.

Against such a backdrop, it is small wonder there is no con-crete advice from my own doctors as to how best to stop taking the progesterone supplements. The participants on the PRISM trial took 400mg of progesterone (or a placebo) as a vaginal suppository twice a day until sixteen weeks. This has been my template for treatment so far. But the published paper only says that treatment was stopped at sixteen weeks. And while I get a reassuring email from the recurrent-miscarriage clinic to tell me that taking aspirin from this point in pregnancy – as opposed to earlier on – is not a problem, when it comes to the progesterone, I'm on my own. If the progesterone *has* been helping, then stopping overnight feels wrong. And if it hasn't, I still feel the need to wean myself off my pharma comfort blan-ket slowly. In the end, I opt for a tapered regimen of my own design, going from two pessaries a day, to one a day, then one every other day, over the course of a week or so. With this gradual withdrawal, I am trying to trick my body into staying pregnant; that it will not notice the difference this way. My body is a wild creature I do not wish to spook.

Progesterone is not the only putative miscarriage treatment for which the evidence has been mixed or non-committal. Major, multi-centre, randomized controlled trials have also found little or uncertain benefit to drugs such as heparin and aspirin. Nick Macklon believes this is due to a fatal flaw in our research approach. 'We use the term recurrent miscarriage as if it were a medical diagnosis, yet there isn't one single medical cause,' he says. It sounds obvious, yet miscarriage research rarely accommodates this. For example – hypothetically – some women may have a blood-clotting disorder, for others a contributing factor could be thyroid dysfunction, while others could be losing multiple, chromosomally abnormal embryos (perhaps because of their age or an over-receptive womb lining). Accordingly, there is unlikely to be a single panacea. Yet scientific studies into preventative treatments tend to recruit participants on the basis that all women who have recurrent miscarriage are the same and are *all* likely to respond to a particular treatment. Lumping together women who have miscarriages in this way, in Professor Macklon's view, is likely to explain why several 'blockbuster' trials of possible treatments have failed to produce convincing evidence. 'The underlying premise, to me, is something that needs to be challenged,' he tells me. His point is that some of these treatments may in fact work for some women, 'but because of the way the study is designed, it comes out as not working overall', he explains. It's a tantalizing – and maddening – prospect for anyone desperate to prevent yet another miscarriage. On the one hand, it means that something there's little evidence for – yet – may in fact help you personally. On the other, it means that something clinically proven may not, in fact, make any difference. The kernel of comfort in all this, I think, is that just because one option doesn't work, doesn't mean nothing will – though, of course, ultimately, we need the nuanced research to take the guesswork out of this.

A related issue is that a lot of the research so far has not made much effort to distinguish between the loss of genetically healthy embryos and those with certain lethal chromosomal abnormalities incompatible with life, where the miscarriage is presumed to be inevitable. As early-pregnancy research fellow Hanine Fourie points out, it's these miscarriages without these changes that really need to be the target for new treatments. 'That's where the modifiable answer might be,' she tells me.

In other words, that's where you might be able to change the outcome of the pregnancy. In a roundabout way, it's possible the PRISM trial into progesterone achieved this distinction to a certain extent – they had an age cut-off of thirty-nine in an attempt to exclude what are more likely to be miscarriages with a chromosomal cause, for example. But it could be that the benefits of progesterone would have been even more pronounced had there been a way to distinguish between euploid and aneuploid miscarriages in the trial.

In recent research that investigated a possible link between bacteria in the vagina and miscarriage, scientists *did* seek to distinguish between chromosomally normal and abnormal losses. Sure enough, they found that while an imbalance in bacteria was associated with miscarrying 'healthy', euploid embryos, the same was not true for women who lost aneuploid pregnancies. This research has opened up the possibility of a relatively simple treatment for some miscarriages: a probiotic – that is, a dose of 'friendly' bacteria.

While the presence of bacteria in the vagina might sound undesirable, and something that only happens should you have an infection, in fact, just like other areas of the body, such as the gut, the vagina has its own 'microbiome' – a community of microbes that live there. 'We have an absolutely essential symbiotic relationship with the bacteria that live in our body,' explains Professor Phillip Bennett, who oversaw the research, which was done by scientists at Imperial College London. 'They are hugely important for our normal function – in fact, if our bodies were sterile, we couldn't survive,' he tells me. 'In reality, we live with millions more bacterial cells than we actually have human cells; there are many more bacterial genes active in our bodies than there are human genes. And what we are now beginning to recognize is that a lot of disease has to do with an imbalance in this normal bacteria.'

In the vagina, a healthy microbiome consists of lots of a

particular type of bacteria called lactobacilli. 'They're good because they create acid, which stops other, less desirable organisms from surviving,' explains Professor Bennett. 'They actually produce specific compounds which are like antibiotics, called bacteriocins, and they kill other bacteria. They also produce anti-inflammatory molecules.' What the Imperial researchers found was that people who miscarried were more likely to have a 'dysbiotic' microbiome; that is, 'lacking in lactobacilli', Professor Bennett tells me.[15] A follow-up study, published in 2021, confirmed that the link existed only when it came to those who were losing chromosomally 'normal' pregnancies. 'It did not apply to people who had aneuploid miscarriages – they actually had quite a low rate of vaginal dysbiosis,' Professor Bennett adds.[16]

Some might find the idea of our bodies being colonized by millions of invisible bacteria wholly unappetizing, but I find it fascinating. To consider that any new life we create potentially also depends on these other, myriad lifeforms within us is humbling, in a way. We humans are more than complicated flesh machines; we are entire ecosystems, diverse and delicate. In the not-too-distant future, Professor Bennett believes, an analysis of the vaginal microbiome will be a routine part of pregnancy monitoring, as normal as blood tests and blood-pressure checks. Although, at the moment, this kind of testing is expensive and it takes several weeks to get the results, a new device is being trialled that can analyse a swab and tell you instantly what bacteria are present. Meanwhile, research is under way to establish whether giving women a probiotic supplement of a particularly helpful kind of lactobacilli, *Lactobacillus crispatus*, can improve the balance of the vaginal microbiome in a pregnancy's favour. In all likelihood, Professor Bennett tells me, probiotic treatment to prevent miscarriage will be trialled before we fully understand how the microbiome supports pregnancy (or not, as the case may be).

Because there's a critical complicating factor here: there were a proportion of people in the Imperial research who had a dysbiotic microbiome but who nonetheless had successful pregnancies. 'So the question becomes, why do some people miscarry and some people not?' says Professor Bennett. 'What we then did was we measured a whole panel of things that are markers of inflammation and what we identified was that people who went on to miscarry also had much higher inflammatory markers than people who didn't.' This, he explains, suggests it's not just the microbiome, but the mother's immune response *to* that microbiome which leads to miscarriage. And unravelling this relationship and the role of the immune system is a much bigger job than being able to identify the particular kinds of bacteria in the vagina and resetting the balance with probiotics. For example, Professor Bennett thinks it may be the case that if there's an unhealthy mix of bacteria in the vagina around the time of conception, the compounds they produce have an effect on the immune cells in the uterus, changing their behaviour and therefore the way the fertilized egg implants and develops. In which case, treatment would have to begin *before* pregnancy, not during. For now, though, this remains a hypothesis. And whatever the answer, it will likely take a long time, and a lot more research, to emerge.

If you've had miscarriages, or trouble conceiving – or both – you may be surprised to hear that our understanding of the role of the immune system is relatively incomplete, because there are already many treatments available privately that claim to target the immune system in order to boost your chances of having a baby. This is a field known as reproductive immunology. The basic idea here is that a hypervigilant immune system may be 'attacking' pregnancies, causing them to fail. Much of the work in this area originates with the American obstetrician Dr Alan Beer, who died in 2006, and once – charmingly – summed up his theory thus: 'Effectively, women become serial killers of their own babies.' A common presumed culprit, for which many seek private testing, are the NK cells, or 'natural killer' cells, that are part of our innate immune system and, among other things, are important for dispatching infected cells and for killing off rogue cells that might otherwise lead to cancer. Popular treatments to dampen down immune activity include steroids or intravenous infusions of intralipids (essentially an emulsion of soybean oil and egg yolk). Both options are thought to suppress inflammation and the activity of natural killer cells.

A few clinics in the UK also offer something called Lymphocyte Immunization Therapy (LIT), in which a woman is given a transfusion of white blood cells from her male partner before she becomes pregnant, in the hope that familiarizing her body with the man's cells in this way will stop the embryo being rejected. It is a little like being vaccinated against your partner, helping the immune system to 'recognize' his cells, but the evidence for it is disputed. In the US, LIT has been banned outside of research trials since 2002 – this was because the Food and Drug Administration considered the therapy to be an 'unsafe' use of a human blood product and because a double-blind, randomized controlled trial published in the *Lancet* had recently shown that it did not, in fact, help recurrent-miscarriage patients.[17] There were also concerns about side effects, ranging from skin welts and rashes to the possibility of triggering autoimmune-type conditions (essentially, sending women's immune systems into overdrive).

Depending on who you talk to, reproductive immunology is either entirely discredited or unfairly maligned. What's certain is it is controversial. As Siobhan Quenby told the *Guardian* newspaper in 2016: 'The two sides actually hate each other. They have to be separated at conferences.' Imperial's Phillip Bennett, for one, is deeply sceptical. He tells me that he often comes across patients who have had their blood tested for

elevated levels of natural killer cells. 'And I've never met someone where it's come out normal – I'm not joking,' he says. 'You
can't have a medical test that's always abnormal; I'm very suspi-
cious of that.' Likewise, while he believes the role of NK cells
in the uterus lining is an important line of enquiry when it
comes to understanding miscarriage, he disputes how valid it is
to test someone's general blood level of circulating NK cells
rather than in the womb specifically (the latter is what happens
at Professor Quenby's research unit in Coventry). 'There's no
scientific logic that the NK cells going around your body are
necessarily anything to do with the NK cell function in the
womb,' he says. 'I think it's a bit of a scam, actually.'

On the other hand, Professor Hassan Shehata, who offers testing for NK cells and other immune-activity markers, along with
steroid treatment for recurrent miscarriage, believes the current
mainstream approach to miscarriage is far too conservative – and
much too quick to dismiss therapies that target the immune
system. Professor Shehata's name is one that comes up again and
again on forums about infertility and miscarriage. He tells me that
he still believes 'immune therapy is going to be the main approach
to recurrent miscarriages' in future and hopes one day to complete a trial to prove, definitively, that steroid therapy works.

The trouble is, the task of getting high-quality evidence to
satisfy those who are understandably sceptical may be getting
harder, not easier. Because the limited evidence for immune
therapies for miscarriage has been overhyped by the private
sector, 'there's almost a prejudice in the medical community',
explains Professor Quenby. 'There are so many poor-quality
studies out there and so few good ones it's very hard to work
out what's what. In order to get a research grant, you need the
promise of peer-review, and so many people are adamantly
against the idea [of reproductive immunology] that it's now
very difficult to come by.' She concludes: 'I'm sure there are
some people who have got an immunological cause of their

miscarriages, but trying to work it out from the current data is impossible.'

What doesn't seem to be in doubt, however, is the importance of the immune system in pregnancy and pregnancy loss – even if we don't fully understand the details. After all, many of the things thought to contribute to recurrent miscarriage, such as anti-phospholipid syndrome and lupus anticoagulant, may be treated with blood-thinning medications, but ultimately they are autoimmune issues; that is, they manifest as clotting disorders but they're caused by a misfiring, overactive immune system. And while we don't yet know the precise ways in which progesterone maintains pregnancy, Professor Coomarasamy tells me, it's thought that the dominant mechanism is probably through some sort of immune-system pathway. Then there's the recent research on how the immune system might be interacting with the microbiome. Professor Bennett concedes it's possible that the current crop of immunological treatments could be working by some mechanism that we don't yet fully understand – 'but in the first place, I'd like to know if they're working at all', he says. 'I think we need to understand much more before we start hitting patients with incredibly powerful drugs like steroids.'

To be caught in the middle of all this, as a patient, can be nothing short of bewildering. Who do you believe? And, above all, what's the harm of trying something? Understandably, many people don't care *how* something works, only whether it does – or not. And everyone's tipping point of cost versus benefit is going to be slightly different. Doctors who adhere firmly to a more conservative approach want to spare you from spending large sums on private treatment that there's no compelling evidence will work and also from unnecessary physical intrusion. But, for all that this is also my own rationalist inclination, I have sometimes felt that subjecting my body to intensive treatment, however needless, would be easier than subjecting my mind to the madness invoked by doing nothing. Recurrent-miscarriage-care nurse Dr Sarah Bailey says she often witnesses the 'constant worry of "Am I getting the right thing?" or "Should I do this?" or "Can I try this?"' in her patients. 'I think if we could standardize the care pathways, then that would go some way to reduce this.'

And offering women nothing is not a neutral position. It risks undermining trust in evidence-based medicine. It throws the door wide open to quackery, pseudo-science, the 'wellness' industry. *It can't hurt* is the frequent refrain of women across the internet describing complicated treatment plans of their own design: high doses of vitamins, such as vitamin D, or CoQ10, or low-dose aspirin. *What have I got to lose?* we ask. *They can't expect me to just sit back and do nothing – can they?* According to end-of-life-care physician Dr David Jarrett, there is a principle in medical ethics – 'often overlooked nowadays' – that medical investigations and treatment should reflect and be appropriate to the life the patient has led. Dr Jarrett uses this concept to question the appropriateness of employing 'the terrifying might of advanced technologies' to artificially prolong the life of an older person 'from an age when cars were a rare sight'.[18] I cannot help wondering if the same question can be asked in the opposite direction, from the opposite end of life's journey. For people like me, raised post-internet, post-IVF, for whom the terrifying might of advanced technology has been a daily reality, is it realistic – ethical, even – to insist on inaction?

As Professor Quenby reflects: 'According to conventional medical dogma, you can only say a treatment works if you're 95 per cent certain that it's effective. And that's fine, but what if you're 90 per cent sure? As an academic, you have to write the paper saying the treatment doesn't work – but if you're a woman who's had a lot of miscarriages, a 90 per cent chance is plenty.' There is, she explains, an ongoing statistical argument about what should count as sufficient evidence. 'I think we're going to see a big change in the way we report trials,' she adds. 'With miscarriage, even if there's a tiny chance it works, in my experience, patients are quite happy to try it. However, the ethical dilemma is that you can explain the risks to a patient and they'll say they don't care. Sometimes they say: "You don't understand – I'd rather die than not have a baby." But as a doctor it's always: "First, do no harm." It's a minefield.'

As someone trying to have a baby, you do not have the luxury of waiting for conclusive long-term data or further research. Currently, I have very little to guide my decisions. Ultimately, I am taking a medication I do not know if I truly need. It is presumed to be very safe – the kind of progesterone I am taking is what's known as 'micronized' progesterone, sometimes referred to as a 'body-identical' hormone. This is because 'it has an identical molecular structure to natural progesterone produced by the ovary and the corpus luteum and then by the placenta in later pregnancy', explains Professor Coomarasamy. 'If you were to do an analysis in the laboratory, you wouldn't be able to tell the difference,' he says. 'That's important because you can change the molecule and sometimes that can make it more potent, but that can also make it risky.' (This proved to be the case for previous synthetic hormones, sometimes given to women in the past.) The kind of progesterone I'm taking is regularly used as part of hormone replacement therapy for women going through the menopause, as well as for transgender women. It is also routinely used in IVF treatment, in the second part of the cycle, up until twelve weeks of pregnancy. But even so, should this pregnancy make it, will I forever be looking back over my shoulder, I wonder? Will I always worry whether future health problems – mine or the baby's – could be traced back to my eagerness to try something, *anything*, to have a baby? There is no easy way to set this anxiety aside.

After a week on my tapered regimen, my supply of progesterone runs out. I can only wait and see what my body will do.

I still cannot feel the baby moving. I attempt to fill the void by compelling myself to perform pregnancy more than I have ever allowed myself to do before. We tell our wider families. I order a bona fide pair of maternity jeans. I join a pregnancy yoga class and, when I go for coffee with some of the other women afterwards, I quite enjoy the accidental impression I give off of being languidly relaxed about this whole pregnancy business. I am, it turns out, the only one who has not booked on to antenatal classes yet. Or had a private gender scan. Or bought a single item of baby paraphernalia. I haven't even made a list. But this, it seems, is read as casual, even a little chaotic, rather than afraid and paranoid. I choose not to correct the interpretation. Somehow, 'four miscarriages' feels like a dangerous incantation to speak in a group of pregnant women you do not know very well. And besides, it's rare that you get to take a holiday from your own personality. For those twenty minutes over herbal tea and cake, I get to be someone else. Someone who wears pregnancy lightly, like an outfit they just decided to throw on one day for fun. For once, I get to be nonchalant, too-cool-for-school, even. I am the Disorganized One. The one whose answer to everything is: 'Oh, I hadn't really thought about it.'

The first flutterings of movement arrive just before our scheduled reassurance scan. Quickening starts as tiny, fizzing bubbles, which within days seem to gather into a rolling wave that crests and churns somewhere beneath my belly button. Sometimes now – increasingly often, in fact – when I lie in bed, I am greeted by a jab from an unseen hand or foot. It feels not unlike the way a panicked heart suddenly thuds against your chest: life punching out at fear the only way it knows how.

9

'It's not a real baby yet'

(March 2020 – 24 weeks pregnant)

'Are you having a boy or a girl, do you know?' The woman behind the counter is smiling at me encouragingly. She has grey-blonde hair and her glasses dangle from a fine chain around her neck.

I shake my head. 'We decided not to find out,' I say, returning her smile.

'Well, I think that's lovely,' she says, as she starts to wrap my purchase in tissue paper. 'So few surprises in life these days, aren't there?'

I continue smiling brightly, simultaneously enjoying the attention while also sensing I am running out of energy for it.

Dan and I have just bought our first item of baby clothing. We have come to the department store straight from a scan. Tomorrow, I will be twenty-four weeks pregnant and this was the deal we made with ourselves. If we got to this point – viability – the point at which it is widely considered a baby has a chance of surviving outside of the womb, we would permit ourselves to buy something. We had discussed doing this after the twenty-week anomaly scan last month, and decided it still felt too soon. But as of tomorrow, whatever happens to us, it will not now be classified as another miscarriage. At the stroke of midnight tonight, this pregnancy becomes a potential person, as far as the law is concerned. Should anything happen now, there is also a reasonable prospect that doctors would try to intervene. From now on, keeping this baby alive is no longer down to my body alone. These are not comforting thoughts exactly, but they are something. They are just enough to buy us twenty minutes among the rails of miniature clothing – the neatly rolled vests stacked inside their plastic multipacks; the doll-sized hats and the shoes the length of my little finger. We choose a simple, white cotton sleepsuit embroidered with rabbits and tiny clusters of stars.

Of course, this milestone we have set for ourselves is an arbitrary one. We know this. I feel neither materially safer than I did yesterday nor that what we stand to lose now is greater than it was this time last week. Trying to ascribe value to human life like this, bisecting it neatly into 'before' and 'after', feels like trying to define the precise point at which winter became spring, when every day has felt just like the one before it. And yet, this is the organizing system we have built around pregnancy. It's inevitable that it infects your thinking, just a little. It undoubtedly shades how we understand and treat miscarriage as a society.

Defining when a foetus becomes a person is not – and has never been – a fixed, easily agreed point. It has shifted around over time, it varies across borders, and changes according to scientific advances, political persuasions, religious beliefs, and individual experience. 'Personhood,' as anthropologist Alma Gottlieb puts it, 'is always a cultural construction'.[1] For example, in early modern England and Colonial America, 'babies were not regarded as fully realized humans at birth, but needed first physical, and later spiritual, guidance and nurture to become fully human', notes the historian Lara Freidenfelds.[2] Accordingly, parents went to great lengths to discourage 'animal' behaviours, including crawling. The Beng people of Côte d'Ivoire traditionally believe that babies are recent reincarnations from the spirit realm and that they need to be persuaded to stay throughout the first years of childhood. Newborns are not considered a person until the umbilical cord falls off.[3] In traditional Jewish law, a distinction is made between foetuses born before and after twenty-one weeks of pregnancy, with the expectation that after twenty-one weeks a foetus should be buried in a Jewish cemetery.[4] In America, unlike the UK, a stillbirth is registered from twenty weeks of pregnancy. Many US states also have foetal homicide laws, which mean a foetus or unborn child can be treated as an individual victim of a crime.

In the UK, our understanding of miscarriage comes from our medico-legal definition of viability, which currently is set at 24 weeks +0 days of pregnancy.* This is the boundary I will cross tomorrow. It was lowered from twenty-eight weeks in April 1991, after medical advances meant more babies born extremely prematurely were surviving. Twenty-four weeks, therefore, became the point from which a death in utero is registered. The legal and clinical definition of miscarriage, as well as the upper limit for abortion, also changed. We have lashed these three ideas together – miscarriage, medicine's ability to keep a baby alive outside of the womb, and the acceptable limit on abortion – and yet thirty years since the threshold last had to be revised, there are signs the relationship is breaking apart once more. Can it hold?

---

* This, too, varies around the world. In Japan, the point of viability was lowered to twenty-two weeks in the 1990s, whereas in many European countries the limit is higher, at twenty-six weeks, on the basis that, although babies might survive from an earlier point, the risk of serious, life-limiting disability remains high.

In 2020, two babies were born before twenty-two weeks who would go on to set new records for survival. Richard Hutchinson, from Wisconsin, in the US, was born at twenty-one weeks and two days. A month later, Curtis Zy-Keith Means, from Alabama, arrived at twenty-one weeks, one day. Both boys defied the odds and celebrated their first birthdays in 2021. These are exceptional stories, of course, and before Richard's birth the global record for premature survival had not changed in thirty-four years. It should also not be overlooked that Curtis was a twin, and his sister C'Asya did not respond to the same treatment and died the day after she was born. In the UK today, generally it is not considered appropriate to offer survival-focused treatment for a baby born before twenty-two weeks. Even so, the point at which survival is considered medically possible has already dropped below the twenty-four-week legal waterline. Between 23 weeks +0 and 24 weeks +6 days of gestation is considered the hinterland of viability, according to the Royal College of Obstetricians and Gynaecologists – an ethically and medically fraught grey-zone in which many factors influence the chance of a baby going on to live a healthy life, such as weight, gender, and various markers of foetal development. (By contrast, after twenty-five weeks, the medical consensus is that treatment should usually be offered.) The boundary of survival, then, is not a bright line, but porous; a fluttering veil that some slip under and some do not. Technological advancements – such as an ongoing project at the University of Michigan to develop an artificial, placenta-like system that can 'breathe' for babies too small and fragile to be put on ventilators[5] – will potentially draw back this curtain still further. What then?

When it comes to both miscarriage and abortion, the border of viability is still rigidly policed, with none of the human nuance that is afforded when it comes to trying to save the lives of the extremely premature. In England, Scotland and Wales, the rules around abortion are enforced not through medical guidelines but via the criminal law. The distinction between miscarriage and stillbirth is a blunt, inflexible cut-off. For those whose much-wanted pregnancies end just before the legal limit of twenty-four weeks, there is no official record of their child's existence, which can be a source of pain and a further disenfranchising of their grief – as can the terminology.* I know several people who do not use the word 'miscarriage' to describe their losses at sixteen, twenty, or twenty-three weeks because it fails to convey what actually happened and what it means to them. (Of course, in its own way, this also obscures the true breadth and depth of the miscarriage experience.)

Some have called for terms such as 'early stillbirth' to be used in place of miscarriage, when a baby is lost in the second trimester, before twenty-four weeks. As for any official change to the threshold for when a miscarriage becomes a stillbirth – or attempting to legally recognize babies lost before twenty-four weeks in some other way – the obvious concern is that implementing any such policy could, unwittingly, threaten access to abortion. This is not a baseless fear. Already, definitions around miscarriage and stillbirth are explicitly set in opposition to each other and used to inform clinical practice around terminations. Clare Murphy, chief executive of the British Pregnancy Advisory Service (BPAS), an independent charity that provides abortion care for the NHS, describes to me a recent warning and clarification from the Department of Health and Social Care that, 'because stillbirth starts at 24 weeks +0, we can only offer abortions up until 23 weeks +6'. While this may not sound like much of a difference, she says, 'there will absolutely be women who can't get an abortion because of that one day'.

---

* However, in summer 2022 it was announced that parents in England would be entitled to a certificate of recognition of their baby after pregnancy loss at any stage of gestation, if – and only if – they would like one.

It is hard to see how perceptions of miscarriage and its significance will truly shift while it is shackled to notions of viability and the legal position on when a life and loss can be recognized, defined in the shadow of abortion law. But as Clare Murphy reflects, 'They don't need to contradict each other.' It might seem a circle that is hard to square, but to truly understand miscarriage, sooner or later you also have to reckon with the history and politics of abortion – and our unresolved anxieties around it.

Here is something you are not supposed to admit if you are a person who has struggled to have a baby: I wasn't always sure I wanted to be a mother. More than that, I have spent most of my life actively afraid of getting pregnant. I have never had to have a termination, but I have taken the morning-after pill three times, once as a teenager and twice at university. The reality of having a baby was very present for me, growing up. I was thirteen when my sister was born – a year before I started my periods and a year before I would let a boy touch me under my clothes for the first time. Before I'd finished puberty, I knew what looking after a baby involved. I knew how to hold a bottle and how to check the temperature of bathwater (on the inside of your wrist, where the skin is thinnest). I saw how tired my mum was, especially when she went back to work. I also saw the looks from strangers in the street if I was ever left to mind the pram alone while we were out shopping; their eyes seeking to extract my shame.

Right through my twenties, I was far more preoccupied with defending my borders against an unplanned pregnancy than I was by the possibility I would not be able to get and stay pregnant. Even once I was married, I remained on the fence about children for a while. When Dan proposed, it was with the promise that our family could look however we wanted it to – a) 2.4 children, b) more cats, or c) none of the above. I don't think it ever occurred to either of us that it might not come down to our choice. Sometimes, I've wondered if it was only after losing that first pregnancy that I knew for certain it was what I wanted.

For all of my teenage and adult life, I had been comfortably convinced of my right not to be pregnant. Unlike previous generations in Great Britain, and many women, still, around the world, I have grown up not knowing a time without access to legal contraception and abortion. The morning-after pill was made available over the counter in this country in 2001, before I had sex for the first time. I was confident but not complacent about any of these things – I understood their importance without knowing what it was like to fight for them; the reflex and inheritance of a third-generation femi-nist. By comparison, when I miscarried – when I wanted to be pregnant but could not make it so – I saw very little in my world that reassured me that my feelings were right or normal. It was confusing. Not least because I would probably once have said that in the first trimester it's not really a baby, it's 'just a bunch of cells'. Had I ever used those exact words myself, or had I just read and internalized them? How did I square my feelings for the six-week heartbeat I'd seen – loved, even – and my identity as a pro-choice woman?

A week after my first miscarriage, Donald Trump was inau-gurated as President of the United States. As I tried to pick up the threads of my old life, unpregnant and seeping sadness, the news cycle felt like it had caught fire. On Trump's first day in the White House, he signed an executive order to reintroduce a ban on federal money going to international aid groups that per-form or provide information on abortions – the so-called 'Mexico City Policy' or global gag rule. Several US states sub-sequently attempted to pass 'heartbeat' bills, which restricted abortion to before cardiac activity can be detected, at around six weeks. A few months later, on the weekend of my second miscarriage, the TV adaptation of Margaret Atwood's *The Handmaid's Tale* aired in the UK. The barbarism of forcing someone to carry a pregnancy acquired a new, highly meme-able visual language. In September that same year, a few weeks after my third miscarriage, Ireland's then Taoiseach, Leo Varadkar, announced that there would be a referendum on the Eighth Amendment to the constitution, which gave a foetus – at any stage of gestation – the same rights as a pregnant woman, and as such represented a near-total ban on abortion in Ireland. With every news story and every miscarriage, the dial on my internal confusion ratcheted up a notch. More noise, more silence.

Having miscarriages did not change the way I felt or thought about reproductive rights. I could find reactionary pieces online in which someone described their volte-face on abortion after pregnancy loss, how it had made them appreciate the 'sanctity of life' for the first time. But that was not how I felt, not exactly. It was more that I was unsure of what to say and how to position my grief. I felt alienated by the language on all sides, unsure of who my allies were.

Throughout this time, in 2017, I started writing more openly about my miscarriages and also engaging with the pregnancy-loss community I found online. The stories I found there and the connections I made with other women and men were – and are – comforting and meaningful to me. Yet, when I first started tip-toeing around this new social media space, I often felt like an impostor, that I was concealing a part of my true self. Again, I ran up against a language barrier. Where others talked apparently unselfconsciously about their 'stars in the sky', their 'heaven babies', or being an 'angel mama', I held myself back, refraining even from using the word 'baby' to refer to my losses. I didn't feel I could make any claim on motherhood, although when others did, I understood the liminal version of maternity they described. There is no word in English for a mother, or parent, without a child. We have widows, widowers, and orphans, but the loss of a child is apparently so unnatural and unspeakable we do not even attempt to accommodate it with language. In this silence, some have turned to the Sanskrit word *vilomah*, which means 'against a natural order' to describe their status as someone who has lost a child, whether during pregnancy or after. This borrowed usage was first suggested in a 2009 essay by Karla Holloway, an English professor at Duke University, North Carolina, and is now frequently used on social media, bringing people together under hashtags such as #vilomah, #vilomahscommunity, and #vilomahhood. More recently, in February 2021, the French politician Mathilde Panot called for 'parange' – a portmanteau of 'parent' and 'ange' (angel) – to be officially adopted into the French language, which also has no native noun for a parent whose child dies.

Then there are the symbols and quotations that attempt to convey the experience of losing a pregnancy to the wider world: stars, flowers, hearts, footprints. This is a realm that emphasizes smallness and borrows liberally from children's fables. Here is A. A. Milne: '"Sometimes," said Pooh, "the smallest things take up the most room in your heart."' And not-quite Tolkien: 'Even the smallest person can change the course of the future.' I felt these things, too, and sometimes I took comfort in their memeification. But I didn't dare use such signifiers myself. Small footprints, tiny hearts. Something in me recoiled from them: it all felt much too close to the language of the pro-life movement. And I was afraid of my grief being misappropriated. I feared being mistaken for the sort of person who pickets abortion clinics, getting in the faces of women who are just trying to get through the day, just doing what they need to do.

Pregnancy loss has a history of being weaponized against reproductive rights. In the UK, US, Canada, Australia, and many other countries, October is designated as baby-loss awareness month – an annual coming-together of activism, fundraising, events, discussion, and writing to highlight issues around pregnancy and infant loss, a broad church that for many participants today encompasses miscarriage, stillbirth, neonatal death, SIDS, ectopic pregnancy, embryo loss, and termination for medical reasons. October 1988 was assigned the first baby-loss awareness month by a joint resolution of the US Congress because 'a greater national effort must be made to provide comfort and assistance to parents who suffer the tragedy of pregnancy loss or infant death'. The resolution was approved by President Ronald Reagan, who, in his accompanying proclamation, couldn't resist adding: 'we can and must do a much better job of encouraging adoption as an alternative to abortion'.[6] He also dropped in an appeal for better care for women afflicted by 'post-abortion syndrome' – a now debunked type of trauma response to having a termination.* That Reagan, who did so much to inflame the debate around reproductive rights, who created the original global gag rule that Trump reinstated, should also be the founding father of a campaigning month for miscarriage and baby loss is uncomfortable for me, to say the least.

While I don't think I ever made overt assumptions about other people's political beliefs just because they spoke in a particular way about their loss, I did hold on to a fear – misplaced, as it would turn out – that being honest about my own views in baby-loss spaces risked rejection. And so, for a time, I felt like a fraud in both conversations: an unwilling double-agent in a culture

---

* High-quality research that has directly compared the psychological responses of women who were able to end their pregnancies with women who tried to access an abortion but were unsuccessful have found no higher rates of trauma symptoms among those who had terminations. For example, one 2016 study found that while two in five women who seek abortions have been found to have one or more symptoms of post-traumatic stress, in many cases this had other triggers, such as a history of rape or sexual abuse. For other women, finding out they were pregnant – or being pregnant – was considered to be the triggering event, rather than the termination. In fact, even among women who did put their distress down to the abortion itself, their answers to researchers' questions suggest this was often rooted in factors such as seeing protestors outside a clinic and the disapproval of others, rather than the procedure or their emotions pertaining to their decision.

war. But I needn't have done. I had fallen for the age-old trickery of a world that divides women and pits them against each other. Good women. Bad women. Women who want children. Women who don't. Women who have miscarriages. Women who need abortions. While it takes a certain leap of empathy for someone who cannot seem to get or stay pregnant to side with someone who desperately wants *not* to be pregnant, our interests are one and the same. Our stories are entwined, like two ancient trees that have grown up and around each other for so long it is hard to know where one begins and the other ends.

For hundreds of years, the English word used to convey the termination of a pregnancy – whether intended or unintended – was one and the same: abortion. It wasn't until 1997 that the UK's Royal College of Obstetricians and Gynaecologists recommended healthcare professionals avoid using the word in cases of spontaneous pregnancy loss. References to 'spontaneous', 'habitual' and 'threatened' abortion still crop up in published academic papers on miscarriage today, though. Now, the clumsy use of these outdated clinical terms – which still sometimes find their way on to medical notes – can still hurt. The pain comes from the threat of being so fatally misunderstood. A gap between your intentions and how others understand them is torn wide open. It pulls on an old injury: the fear that you lost this pregnancy because of something you did.

But the capacity these words have to wound only really exists in a context in which women *can* choose to end a pregnancy, in which it is a legitimate possibility. By contrast, as the historian Leslie Reagan has identified, in the 1940s and 1950s the label 'spontaneous abortion' was used in mainstream magazines, blaring from headlines on health features about miscarriage in a way that would be deemed unthinkably insensitive now.[7] Perhaps, before abortion was legalized, the word had yet to be laden with the stigma and political baggage it now carries. Back when no one could choose an abortion, they were sometimes passed off as miscarriages (because, of course, abortions still happened, legal or not), while miscarriages could be referred to as abortions without it meaning something a woman wanted or made happen. In this way, the fluidity of the word represented protection, not pain – 'natural' or unintended pregnancy loss was a shield that women could hide behind. (Sadly, for some women who get pregnant unintentionally, this tactical deployment of the word 'miscarriage' may once again become a necessity. In the aftermath of the US Supreme Court's decision to overturn Roe *v.* Wade, America's uneasy legal arrangement that was supposed to protect the right to abortion, some reproductive-rights campaigners advised that if someone needed medical attention after an illegally obtained abortion they should protect themselves from prosecution by telling healthcare workers they'd had a miscarriage, the two things being clinically indistinguishable, requiring the same medications.)

But, historically, this ambiguity created by a lack of legal abortion has had ramifications for the medical treatment of miscarriage. Although there was an increased interest in early pregnancy and improving the chances of the unborn in the early part of the twentieth century, especially after the huge loss of life in the First World War, doctors refrained from asking too many questions of patients who miscarried in case they put themselves in a difficult position with regards to 'professional secrecy' should they suspect someone had illegally induced a miscarriage. Therefore 'doctors and the state were able to observe the effects, rather than the causes, of pregnancy loss, and even then, only partially', writes the historian Dr Rosemary Elliot.[8] It also meant they had no way of reliably assessing the true prevalence of miscarriage. I can't help wondering, how much further on would our current understanding be if we'd had legal abortion sooner? And, for that matter, how much blurrier that understanding might become, now that America has turned back the clock on reproductive rights?

Even in this country, the decisions we make around abortion provision continue to impact miscarriage care. At a purely clinical level, the treatment required to manage a missed miscarriage or a termination – the medication, the surgery – is often one and the same. Yet because one thing is governed by medical guidelines while the other is controlled by criminal law, they are kept apart, treated as discrete concerns. Because abortion care is still stained as 'political' rather than purely medical, it has been hived off and, for the most part, kept separate from NHS services, outsourced to charities and independent providers, rather than being done within NHS hospitals or clinics. 'This segmentation of women's reproductive healthcare is not helpful,' says Clare Murphy, of the British Pregnancy Advisory Service (BPAS). 'Eighty per cent of abortions are no longer provided in the NHS, they're provided in the independent sector, such as by BPAS or Marie Stopes,' she tells me. 'In some ways, this has been the best and worst thing for abortion in the UK. At one level, it's brilliant because women come to us and they get a dedicated, compassionate, non-judgemental service. But it also means it's taken out of the NHS and it doesn't sit alongside all these other issues in women's reproductive healthcare. It's somehow seen as a completely separate, stigmatized issue in women's lives. But the flipside is you do have an organization that is dedicated to this area of women's care. You could argue that, in many respects, this has meant we have a great abortion service, but we have a patchier miscarriage service, which doesn't have a clinical champion in quite the same way.'

This compartmentalization divides resources and expertise, argues Murphy. And miscarriage care has suffered as a result. For example, for women who have second-trimester miscarriages, who need or want surgery, 'you don't necessarily have the surgical skills in the NHS to deal with them, whereas you do in the independent sector', Murphy tells me. 'If what we had was a properly funded abortion *and* miscarriage service, for one thing women having second-trimester miscarriages might get more choice,' she adds. As it stands, women who have a late missed miscarriage or who need a surgical termination for medical reasons are often told they will have to go to a BPAS or Marie Stopes clinic. While independent-sector clinics have well-developed pathways for this kind of loss to reflect that this was a wanted pregnancy, telling someone they have to go to a separate abortion clinic still has the potential to add a layer of judgement, shame, and trauma where there needn't be one. It is 'beyond cruel', in the words of Laura Gray, a lecturer, who made the difficult decision to end her pregnancy after finding out at sixteen weeks that her daughter had a serious medical complication. She was told that the NHS couldn't provide surgery, only a medical induction. 'I'm very pro-choice and would never judge anyone for the decisions they make – but to ask someone who is ending their very-much-wanted pregnancy due to medical reasons to go to an abortion clinic can't be right,' she says.

Treating all women under the umbrella of a neutral NHS service, on the other hand, could exorcize this spectre of moral judgement. 'There are so many ways these services could, clinically, go hand in hand,' says Clare Murphy. 'You'd have to recognize that women coming into abortion and miscarriage services will have different psychological needs,' she adds – though, again, such a service could create room for a greater degree of emotional nuance. 'Despite the nature of the intervention, women's feelings about it might be very different,' Murphy points out. 'While abortion can be a very straightforward decision and not always a tragedy, for lots of women it has been a difficult and sad decision. And there will be women seeking care for miscarriage who just want to get on with their lives.'

But there are subtler consequences, too, of 'pro-life' anxieties and dogma, such as stymieing scientific research, including – with not a little irony – research into pregnancy loss. While we might not like to think about it, donated embryonic and foetal tissue is important for furthering medical understanding, not only of pregnancy, but all kinds of conditions, from cancer and HIV to genetic causes of blindness. In this country, since 1999, after someone has decided they wish to terminate a pregnancy, they may be asked if they wish to contribute to the Human Developmental Biology Resource, a tissue bank for researchers. No money exchanges hands and the idea is not suggested or discussed while someone is still making their decision, so as not to influence them either way. The scientists who, in 2021, were able to map and observe the behaviour of the cells of an embryo during the 'black box' period of gastrulation for the very first time – beyond the usual fourteen-day time limit – were able to do so because of an embryo that was donated following a termination. But not all countries allow this. In 2019, Donald Trump's government made it effectively impossible for scientists to use this kind of donated foetal tissue in their research – the US's National Institutes of Health, which is the largest public funder of biomedical research in the world, was no longer permitted to back projects that did. Under President Biden's administration, the most recent restrictions were reversed, but this will not immediately undo the damage. Meanwhile, 'personhood' laws, such as the one passed in the US state of Indiana that insists on the burial or cremation of foetal tissue after miscarriage and abortion, regardless of a woman's wishes, also rule out the possibility of tissue being donated to medical research.

Here in the UK, where abortion is both legal and widely accepted, recent anti-abortion campaigning efforts have shifted focus – some might say cynically – to argue against 'discriminatory' abortion on the basis of suspected disability. In particular, objections have been raised to advances in prenatal screening such as non-invasive prenatal testing (NIPT), a blood test that looks at DNA from the placenta to more accurately assess the risk of certain genetic conditions. In 2021, this started to be rolled out across the NHS, but it has been fought all the way by groups such as Right To Life, as well as campaigns such as Don't Screen Us Out.* The debate tends to centre around the fact that this kind of testing looks for trisomy 21, better known as Down's syndrome. But what is often overlooked is that NIPT has the potential to reduce the number of miscarriages that happen every year as a result of more invasive screening techniques that women otherwise have to rely on, such as taking a sample from the placenta or amniotic fluid. And yet, the 'pro-life' movement doesn't seem all that interested in these potential lives.

None of this is simple. There are only shades of grey. Perhaps outdated attitudes to disability and unfair perceptions of Down's syndrome have shaded how some people are counselled when a prenatal diagnosis is made. But perhaps more to the point is the uncertainty inherent in any such a diagnosis; what medics are unable to tell people for certain about the future health of their baby, when the consequences of a condition exist on a spectrum. At the same time, blunt statistics about the high proportion of Down's syndrome pregnancies that are terminated each year do not reflect individual medical nuance, overlapping physical complications, or hard realities about a parent's resources. And what of the overwhelming fear someone may have of another miscarriage or stillbirth? This is almost never mentioned – and yet for babies diagnosed with Down's syndrome or the two other, rarer, trisomies that we screen for, the risk of this happening rises substantially.† There are so

---

* The idea that introducing NIPT will lead to fewer babies born with Down's syndrome is not necessarily factual, however. Data from pilot schemes in NHS hospitals so far suggests that this kind of screening doesn't significantly increase the number of cases of Down's syndrome detected, or the number of subsequent terminations as a result; it just makes the information-seeking process less invasive.
† When it comes to the other two, rarer trisomies we screen for – Edwards' and Patau's syndromes – around 70 per cent of pregnancies diagnosed with these conditions at twelve weeks go on to end in miscarriage or stillbirth. Where Down's syndrome is diagnosed, an estimated 30 per cent of pregnancies will end in spontaneous loss after twelve weeks, according to the Down's Syndrome Association.

many reasons someone might not feel able to continue with a pregnancy after Down's syndrome or another genetic condition has been diagnosed, reasons which have nothing to do with the pursuit of genetic perfection or believing that such children are lesser.* Would I be able to continue with this pregnancy if a serious condition is diagnosed – even a potentially non-fatal condition – if it conferred an even higher risk of miscarrying than I have already? What would that do to my already fragile mental health? This is the fear that stalked me in the gap between our twelve-week scan and getting the results of our own screening test, and again ahead of our twenty-week 'anomaly' scan. But there was another dread that shadowed it. Should this baby be seriously unwell, would I have the strength to opt for a termination if I thought it would, ultimately, spare them from pain and suffering? If called upon, could I put their best interests ahead of my own desire for a child? It is easy to think you know your 'moral' position on such matters, especially if what you want, more than anything, is to have a baby. But I do not think anyone can truly know what they would do until they have lived it – even then, they only know what was right for them.

The difference that access to safe, legal termination makes to the scoresheet of ongoing human life cannot be measured as tidily as anti-abortion campaigners claim. For every life – or potential life – you force into being with laws, restrictions, and scaremongering, another might be lost in the infinite, immeasurable maelstrom of cause and effect. More might be miscarried, needlessly. Thousands might be lost to illness and disease that we never find cures for. Others might never be created in the first place.

---

* When this is how the debate is so often framed, it's little wonder that those who have terminations for medical reasons rarely discuss it openly – even though this kind of pregnancy loss is more common than stillbirth, with at least 5,000 occurring every year.

An all-but-forgotten detail in the story of the world's first
IVF baby, Louise Brown, is that her parents, Lesley and John,
had to sign a document agreeing that if prenatal testing revealed
any sort of genetic abnormality, they would terminate the pregnancy.[9] Lesley and John's remarkable journey to parenthood
was told to the world through a syndication deal with the *Daily
Mail*. Their story wasn't framed as a tale of terrifying, unnatural
technology or doctors 'playing God', but as the very human
struggle of two ordinary, working-class people who simply
wanted a family. As the sociologist Katie Dow has argued, this
shaped the global narrative around IVF right from the start,
paving the way for its normalization.[10] What if policymakers,
'pro-life' campaigners, and more conservative sections of the
media had decided that what the Browns and their doctors were
doing was morally unacceptable – not least because of the clause
requiring an abortion in certain circumstances? Inconvenient as
it might be to those who claim to champion the sanctity of life,
availability of safe termination does not only help women who
wish not to be pregnant – it helps those who really, really do.

It's not only the pro-life version of events that leaves out pregnancy loss, however. Miscarriage has been equally inconvenient to the pro-choice narrative, at times. As the Canadian writer
and feminist Alexandra Kimball has identified, infertility and
pregnancy loss have, historically, been overlooked by the feminist movement. The rallying cries of the 'right to choose', 'my
body, my choice', and 'every child a wanted child' represent
'an exclusive mandate, assuming that every woman who
wanted a child was capable of having one', she writes.[11] Like
me, after her miscarriages Kimball felt 'not just invisible to the
ideology I'd grown up with, I felt forsaken'.[12] Throughout the
1970s and 1980s, influential feminists made plain their revulsion
at the idea of assisted reproduction, apparently objecting to the
intrusion of male-dominated medicine into something that

was sacredly, intuitively feminine. It's an attitude that never really went away for a certain kind of feminism.

Columnists arguing for fewer restrictions on abortion pills continue to describe early pregnancies as 'a bunch of cells', 'blobs', 'not much more than a fertilized egg', echoing the hurtful ways people seek to minimize your feelings after a miscarriage or unsuccessful IVF cycle, while surrogacy in particular is treated with suspicion. *'Surrogacy snaps the mother–baby bond in two – we should not celebrate it as progress'* condemned the headline of one think-piece for the left-wing magazine the *New Statesman* in 2021, with no heed paid to surrogacy sometimes being the last or only option for some infertile women, as well as for gay men and some trans people.

There is a context, of course, to feminism's relative silence on miscarriage. Grief over pregnancy loss has only emerged as a dominant experience now that women have greater control of their fertility. As the historian Leslie Reagan has argued, the significance of miscarriage shifted throughout the twentieth century 'from hazard to blessing to tragedy'. It is almost impossible for us now to imagine the tyranny of being able to do so little to prevent pregnancy; how for many a miscarriage could well have been seen as a blessing.

But this is only a partial excuse, one part of a much bigger story. For many women, throughout history, the right to have a child has been as central to overturning their oppression as the right to choose not to. From the abysmal rates of stillbirth and infant and child mortality among enslaved people in America – estimated to have been double those of the entire US population at the time – to government-sponsored forced sterilization of Black and indigenous women in the US and Canada throughout the twentieth century, the right to reproduce has not been a given for non-white women. Indeed, the origins of the fight for reproductive rights cannot be disentangled from white supremacy. The first feminist ambassadors for legal contraception and abortion, such as Margaret Sanger, the founder of Planned Parenthood in the US, and the UK's Marie Stopes, were motivated, at least in part, by eugenics.* During feminism's first wave, the case for family planning was often justified in terms of racial purity and curtailing the fertility of 'defectives' and 'human weeds': the poor, the disabled, Jews, and people of colour. 'Every child a wanted child' – but wanted by whom? In Australia, child-removal policies, which sanctioned mixed-race Aboriginal and Torres Strait Islander children being taken away from their parents to be adopted by white families, placed in care, or sent to board at schools far from home, were in place until 1969. In 2020, there were allegations that immigration detention centres in the US had carried out forced, unnecessary hysterectomies on women. A senate committee on human rights in Canada reported at least one case of forced sterilization as recently as 2019. Meanwhile, American research has suggested that Black women may be twice as likely to be infertile as white women, while UK data from the Human Fertilisation & Embryology Association published in 2021 suggests that people from ethnic minority backgrounds are less likely to have a baby after fertility treatment, with Black women having the lowest success rates, raising questions about the treatment and care they receive. Yet feminism has overwhelmingly privileged the concerns of the white, straight, fertile, middle-class women it assumes as its norm – and that has typically meant contraception and abortion. Sometimes to the exclusion of all else.

The tweet hit my eyes like stinging salt water: 'STOP TRYING TO MAKE "ECTOPIC PREGNANCIES ARE BABIES TOO" A THING.' It went on: 'If you have never treated a woman with a belly full of blood from an ectopic you should shut the fuck up and sit down and learn before you get someone killed.' The blast

---

* Stopes infamously sent a volume of fan-girl love poetry to Hitler.

came from a medical doctor and feminist campaigner I admire and usually agree with. But this hurt. I was a year on from my fourth miscarriage and had recently started trying to conceive again. By then, I knew more than a few women who considered their ectopic pregnancies to be babies they never got to meet. The tweet wasn't aimed at me, personally; it was drawing attention to horrifying instances of some Catholic hospitals in the US apparently refusing to give women diagnosed with an ectopic pregnancy the drug methotrexate, based on a belief that to do so represents an unacceptable severing of sacred life. Methotrexate kills rapidly dividing cells to end an out-of-place pregnancy. An ectopic pregnancy is never viable, but left untreated it can cause a catastrophic haemorrhage that risks a woman's life. And yet even this is not enough to exempt it from hard-line positions on abortion. In 2022, Missouri legislators introduced a bill that would make it a crime to treat an ectopic pregnancy, while in 2019, a bill in Ohio tried to insist that in cases of ectopic pregnancy, doctors 'reattach' the embryo in the right place in the womb. No such operation exists. As Professor Daniel Grossman, a public health researcher in abortion and contraception, explained at the time, it is 'pure science fiction'.

I have not had an ectopic pregnancy. But, after my fourth miscarriage, I was investigated for a suspected molar pregnancy — where the fertilization of an egg goes awry and there is either too much or too little genetic information for an embryo to develop; instead, a mass of abnormal cells starts to form. Sometimes, rarely, this can become invasive and requires an approach akin to cancer treatment. Like an ectopic pregnancy, a molar pregnancy is never viable either. But that does not mean its loss hurts less. Being told that what I thought was an embryo could potentially be a clump of cancerous cells invading my womb did nothing to un-conceive the baby I had in my mind, if not in body. I composed and deleted reply after reply to that tweet. But in the end, I did indeed 'just shut the fuck up'.

Sometimes, the cost of telling certain stories feels too high; some truths too dangerous. When we're looking at where silences around miscarriage come from, it's not only self-censorship, it's how we are censored when our stories don't serve another – equally important – narrative. And yet why can't we have both? Why should we have to choose between life-saving medical treatment, reproductive freedom, *and* recognition for what a nascent lifeform can mean to us? I've seen the argument made by pro-choice advocates that, because ectopic pregnancies are never viable, we should stop calling them pregnancies altogether – a sentiment I can't help finding hurtful. It is profoundly depressing to me that in order to protect a woman's basic human rights, we have to deny the humanity – even the existence – of an early pregnancy altogether.

There are signs things are changing. The ultimately successful campaign to repeal the Eighth Amendment in Ireland, making abortion legal before twelve weeks, did not fight its case on these terms. Rather than directly contradicting a notion that life begins at conception, it focused on the many, many ways enshrining this belief in law becomes inhumane. Alongside the stories of women who didn't want to be pregnant, the repeal campaign told the stories of women who did, but who were punished by the law all the same: miscarrying women; women told their baby had a fatal condition who were forced to travel to England to end the pregnancy compassionately, rather than see their newborn suffer and die within hours. The campaign emphasized and amplified stories like that of Savita Halappanavar, who died while on holiday in Galway, in 2012, after being denied treatment as she miscarried at seventeen weeks pregnant on the basis that to do so would break the law. Even though Savita was told her baby would not survive, doctors refused to induce her or operate because there was still a faint foetal heartbeat – by the time the baby had died in utero days later, and doctors acted, Savita had contracted an infection. She died of sepsis twenty-four hours later. As well as laying bare the cruelty of the law, such stories confounded an enduring myth around abortion: that women who do it, or those who support it, do so because they undervalue human life. If anything, the opposite is true – something women are increasingly finding ways to articulate.

Kathryn Mann, an artist, had an abortion when she found out she was pregnant early on in a new relationship, not long after the breakdown of her previous marriage. Like around 85 per cent of abortions in the UK, it was done with medication rather than surgery. Kathryn explains: 'The night before taking the mifepristone tablet, I spoke to the apple-pip-sized, five-week-old embryo growing inside me and explained why I had to end the pregnancy.' Today, she counts this loss alongside the five miscarriages she would go on to have. 'I know I made the right decision at the time, but as with each subsequent loss, I held them for every moment of their existence, so I can also acknowledge the person they might've been.'

We all have our own ideas about when life begins and what is best for our children or would-be children. Which brings us back to viability. While we measure miscarriage against abortion, against medical viability, it will always be seen as lesser. By definition – in the UK and many countries around the world – a miscarriage is not the loss of a person. For some, this feels like the shape of it: their grief is for something intangible and nameless, rather than for a someone. But that is not everyone's experience. For some, their loss is a child they named, dressed, held, and commemorated with pictures and, perhaps, a funeral. Would it really be so unworkable for the law to find ways to reflect this difference – to record these lost lives, or almost-lives – while leaving abortion provision unchanged? Or to look at it another way, perhaps this is a further argument for why abortion should be governed by medical guidelines, with the nuance, pragmatism and human kindness that allows, rather than crudely enforced by criminal law.

There are many who argue that the only logical, moral response to recent medical advances in keeping pre-term babies alive is to, once again, lower the agreed definition of viability along with the upper limit on abortion. This was attempted as recently as November 2021 in the UK. Proponents of such changes often question how it can be right that 'in one room of a hospital, doctors could be working to save a baby born alive before 23 weeks whilst, in another room, a doctor could perform an abortion that would end the life of a baby at the same age'.[13] But this is disingenuous. It is a fundamental mistake to assume that the woman ending her pregnancy ascribes a different value to that life than the woman in the 'other room' of the hospital praying doctors can resuscitate her baby. To bring down the abortion time-limit on the grounds that babies survive from this point also overlooks the incredibly complicated medical realities of this stage of gestation and the difficult decisions many parents have to make if their baby is born in the grey-zone. Viability is not the same as a baby being guaranteed to survive independently. A premature baby's chance of survival, or avoiding serious disability, doesn't catch up with the odds for a baby born full term until thirty-four weeks. No one invokes the sanctity of life to argue that the parents of a baby born at twenty-three weeks must agree to invasive treatment at all costs. No one seems to see any inherent moral dilemma in the different approach of two cancer patients, treated by the same hospital, one choosing to try everything and anything they can, the other opting for palliative care. So why can't we accept the same degree of nuance when it comes to life in the womb? I don't think it is unreasonable or illogical to believe that life begins at conception. I also don't think this has to be incompatible with supporting abortion.

At home, I put the rabbit sleepsuit, still in its tissue-paper membrane, safely away at the bottom of the wardrobe in the room we have not yet decorated as a nursery. I check my messages. My dad's flight has landed. He's coming over from France to stay with us and tomorrow we're all going out to dinner for my grandma's birthday. It's been a strange week. Cases of a novel coronavirus they are calling Covid-19 are rising in the UK. Three people over here have died from it. The stock market wobbled. Interest rates have been slashed. 'Recession' say the news bulletins. 'Herd immunity.'

The next day, I drive the three of us – four if you include the baby – out into the Peak District to dinner. The roomy dress I'd bought just a few weeks ago now pulls tight across my stomach. It's already dark when we set off and I am a nervous driver, but I offer to do it because I need the practice. Driving, somehow, feels integral to the person I am hoping to become. I want to be the kind of woman who can drive on the other side of the road on family holidays abroad without giving it a second thought, car packed to the rafters with bodyboards, bikes, kids, and dogs. I want to be able to launch solo rescue missions at midnight for teenagers stranded at parties and music festivals. I want to be able to navigate strange cities for university visits, and beyond.

Ten minutes away from the restaurant, I wait to emerge at a junction, which sits underneath a railway arch. The maw of a giant's lair. I crane my neck right, then left, then right again, then go. But I don't give it quite enough gas, and the car stalls. We're only stranded for a moment, but it's enough. The noise and the impact are the same. I can't tell where one begins and the other ends. It sounds heavy. It feels loud. I'm shunted forwards in my seat. My chest constricts. It takes me a minute to understand that the van behind us has gone into the back of our car.

'It's OK, it's OK,' Dan is saying.

My hands go to my stomach. My mind burns white-hot with panic.

10

'Better safe than sorry'

(March 2020 – 24 weeks pregnant)

In the seconds after the car accident – little more than a prang, really – my whirring brain falls blank and silent. It turns out, when I am truly scared, when there is an obvious, material reason to fear for the baby, like a van crunched up against our bumper, I no longer feel hyperactively worried: I feel nothing.

I sit like a statue while Dan exchanges details with the van driver, who is panicked and apologetic. My hands remain clamped to my stomach. I close my eyes and try to divine movement below the surface. Had the baby been moving before? I'd been concentrating on driving, so I cannot be certain either way. At some point, it is decided that the car is dented, but safe. Dan says he will drive us from here. As I get out and walk around to the passenger seat, I feel exposed in the cold night air. My dress is a pale cotton button-down thing, the hem skimming the top of my winter boots. In the headlights, I am lit up like a ghost.

We carry on to the restaurant. Dan asks if I want to go and get checked out, for peace of mind, but something in me resists. Partly, this is because I think I know I am fine. Partly, it is because if we don't go, no one can tell me otherwise. When we arrive, I go straight to the bathroom. There is no blood. No other 'loss from below', as the midwives put it. My lungs let go of some air I hadn't realized they'd been holding on to. At the table, I sip some sparkling water and nibble a piece of bread, the butter sharply salted, and the baby fizzes awake. As they stretch and roll against my insides, I reach for Dan's hand, and wait for a gap in the conversation to whisper to him that the baby is moving. Their kicks stay reassuringly strong all evening. Tomorrow, I will phone the maternity unit just to be sure, but for now I am OK. We are OK. Tomorrow, the midwife I speak to will agree that there doesn't seem to be any cause for concern, but to call again or come in if I'm worried. Tomorrow, Dad will fly home. We will hug at the airport, as normal. But the day after tomorrow, the prime minister will give a press conference. The day after tomorrow, vulnerable people, including those who are pregnant, will be instructed to stay at home for their own safety. A week after that, the whole of the UK will go into lockdown to try to stop this new virus from swamping our hospitals. And, much later, we will look back and wonder at how it could have all felt so normal, just days away from catastrophe.

The initial days of my confinement are softened by activity: batch-cooking, arranging deliveries, and cancelling plans. Dan, who is a criminal barrister and still travelling in and out of Manchester for work, takes his temperature every day with the thermometer I used to use to monitor for signs of ovulation. We are unsure what is safe and what is paranoia. We take extra precautions. When Dan gets home, he changes and showers before we touch. I clean door handles and light switches with bleach. I read the official guidance from the Royal College of Obstetricians and Gynaecologists, over and over: *'There is no evidence to suggest an increased risk of miscarriage.' 'Pregnant women are still no more likely to contract coronavirus than the general population.'*

Overnight, all my nebulous anxieties about what might happen to this pregnancy have solidified into something concrete. The task of keeping this baby safe feels heavier with every passing day. And it feels more difficult now to dismiss my fear as simply hypothetical, based on our past experience, not our current reality. Now, I can plot my anxiety against the graphs tracking the daily number of reported cases, hospital admissions, and deaths. Rising, rising, rising. Then the newspapers start to report the first deaths of pregnant women. When those front pages land, I can barely look at them. The screen-grabbed pictures from wedding days; the details of how many days old their babies are – motherless. I have worried that this baby might not make it every day since I first took a pregnancy test – perhaps even before that, as I willed them into being. Now, for the first time, it occurs to me that I could die, too. After a week of lockdown, I wake in the night feeling hot, my throat scratchy and constricted. This is it, I think – I've caught it. I have barely been outside for a fortnight, though I did get my hair cut a few days before lockdown was announced. *What a stupid, unnecessary risk*, I think, staring up at the ceiling. *We could die. And for what? Split ends and a few grey hairs*. In the morning, though, I feel fine. *Heartburn*, I tell myself. It seems obvious in the rational light of day.

The world shrinks. On Saturdays, I allow myself to look at a pregnancy app, to confirm that another week has been checked off: 25 weeks +0 . . . 26 weeks +0. The fear is intense. Sometimes, it takes up so much space that even the slightest additional intrusion feels intolerable. I silence all notifications and delete social media accounts from my phone. Another thought or question and my mind will break open like an egg. Because, mixed in with the fear, there is also a secret sadness. A guilty longing for things I will not now get to do: a 'last' holiday as a couple, wearing a maternity dress at my brother's now-postponed wedding, making and meeting new 'mum friends' for coffee. Recurrent miscarriage has sometimes felt like being swindled by a fairy-tale villain – a fate devised by a sly genie. I had naively wished only to get pregnant and Rumpelstiltskin had taken me at my literal word. I would get pregnant again, and again, and again. Only, now that I have grown wiser and been more specific with my wish – to stay pregnant for long enough, to have a baby – the trickster has found another way to subvert our bargain. But this feels like an unspeakably selfish way to think, in the circumstances. I cannot admit it to anyone.

I instruct myself to be grateful. I am grateful for our house. For our jobs. For each other. Above all, I am grateful I am pregnant. I am grateful I am relatively far along. Sometimes this works, at other times it only loops back into more guilt. 'Just think how much worse it could be,' Dan and I take turns to say to each other. 'Just imagine . . .' Only, I do not really need to imagine. The other life we could have been living is painfully present. I walk around with her all day, this other me, who had a fifth miscarriage and now doesn't know if it feels safe to try to conceive again. Some days, she is only a few weeks pregnant and is not allowed into the hospital for extra reassurance scans, as units are trying to limit the number of people around, to protect other patients and NHS staff. Occasionally, my shadow-companion has just been told she's had a missed miscarriage, at a scan she was asked to attend alone, the news broken by a masked midwife who cannot hug her – or even hold her hand.

Maternity care has been an unwitting casualty of the pandemic, as the wagons are circled around our hospitals. A postcode patchwork of new rules and restrictions has been established. Women are expected to attend routine scans and appointments alone, and in many cases cannot have someone with them on labour wards until the later, 'active' stages. Home births are being restricted or advised against. Visitors are strictly prohibited on postnatal wards. Health visitors and midwives are encouraged to contact new parents remotely, rather than see them face to face. Parents of babies in neonatal intensive care cannot visit their fragile newborns together – or sometimes even at all. In all of this, though, miscarriage and infertility patients remain something of an afterthought. It takes weeks for specific guidance to miscarrying women even to be included in the official advice on pregnancy and Covid-19. Fertility treatment has been stopped altogether virtually overnight. This, too, functions as a kind of pregnancy loss. Although you could never know whether that particular cycle would have been the one that worked, even just the chance of being pregnant in two weeks' time is taken away from you. That version of your future is stopped, abruptly, irretrievably. The vanishing act that's at the heart of all grief.*

My due date is still several months away, so I am not permitting myself to think about the practicalities of a pandemic birth just yet. The closest I get is to hope that things will be going back to something approaching normal by then. I find it much harder to put aside my guilty thoughts about what is happening to people who have been less lucky in pregnancy than we have been – so far – this time. More than ever, I am conscious that we are separated by the flimsiest of veils; another fate only ever a few millimetres away.

People are talking about a Covid 'baby boom'. Stuck at home, what else would couples do other than have lots and lots of sex,

---

* Indeed, one small study from America, where treatment was similarly affected by the pandemic, suggested that withdrawal of fertility treatment – and therefore the opportunity to become pregnant – was experienced as equivalent to the loss of a child by 22 per cent of people.

which of course always leads to babies in nine months. These predictions leave me with a knotted feeling under my ribs. I am offended by the idea that anyone would decide to make a baby out of sheer boredom. Or perhaps it is the idea they *could* that offends me; that it comes so easily to some people. To me, the jokes feel jarring, like an attempt to add canned laughter to scenes from a dystopian drama. More than ever, I find myself questioning what kind of world I will be bringing a child into. In this new light, everything is laid bare: the competence (or not) of our politicians. The preparedness (or not) of our health-care system. The capaciousness (or not) of our social safety nets. How vulnerable we are. How powerless.

Yet still, the baby-boom talk persists. Sometimes, this makes me feel like a Covid Cassandra, convinced the jovial predictions must be wrong.* More often, I suspect that I am just being a kill-joy; that perhaps it's me who is detached from reality, made unduly pessimistic by our medical history. Even so, it feels so at odds with the message that is hammered into women and pregnant people at every opportunity: *Better safe than sorry*. And surely nobody feels very safe right now?

After several weeks of isolation, I get all dressed up to go to an appointment at the hospital. I put on eyeliner, lipstick, and real shoes – not slippers, not wellies – for the first time in what feels like for ever. It is too warm for the long, grey jumper I have worn to all my appointments so far so, superstitiously, I stuff it into my handbag instead. The roads are eerily quiet and

---

* Eventually, it'll be shown that birth rates declined during the pandemic. The number of babies born nine months or more after the emergence of Covid fell sharply in the UK, as well as in Europe, parts of Asia, and in the US. What's more, a study led by Dr Sara White, a senior research fellow in women's and children's health at King's College London, showed that almost three quarters of couples (72 per cent) who had been actively planning a pregnancy between January and July 2020 postponed their plans. The reasons they gave for this were not only fear of catching the virus itself, but also anxiety around its effects on antenatal care.

the motorway, when we hit it, feels uncomfortably fast from
the passenger seat. So much of what was once normal already
feels unfamiliar and alien. I drink in the sights like a tourist. The
closed retail parks and shuttered drive-throughs. The railway
lines into the city, without trains. I notice everything: every
roundabout, every empty car dealership. All of it quenching a
need that I didn't know I had.

At the hospital, as per the new rules, Dan doesn't come in
with me. Instead, he waits in the car, as a burly security guard
on the maternity-unit door checks my name off on a clip-
boarded list. Today, I am here for the full works: a scan,
followed by bloods with the midwife, and then a check-in with
the consultant. I can feel the baby ferreting around as I sit in the
waiting room, so, for once, I am not unduly worried about the
scan. Even so, I wish I wasn't alone. I ask the masked sonographer if I can video-call Dan, but they say no. And I don't push
it. At least he was here for the other scans, I tell myself – while
also resenting that my mind reaches so reflexively for the empty
consolation of 'at leasts'. I thought we'd left those behind: *At
least you can get pregnant . . . At least it was early.*

In the doctor's office, I perch on the wipe-clean examination
bed at the far end of the long, oblong room, while the consultant sits at his computer, near the door. To make myself heard
from this far away, through my surgical mask, I have to project
my voice, like a bad stage actor. 'No, no family history of
diabetes,' I enunciate. 'No, no headaches. No blurred vision.'
Although everything is fine, I am at the hospital for nearly two
hours, all in. In the second of the two waiting rooms, I have no
phone signal, so cannot update Dan. When I finally emerge
from the hospital into the car park, each vehicle I pass is occu-
pied by a man in the same hunched pose: head bowed, phone in
hand.

While the schedule of my hospital appointments has continued unaffected, the same cannot be said of the checks with

the local midwife, who I am supposed to see in between. I know I have not been in since eighteen weeks. Or was it sixteen weeks? Whatever it is, it feels like too long a gap. At the same time, I wonder if they've not contacted me yet because it's safer for me not to go into the GP's surgery just now. It is hard to know what is right, what is necessary. In the end, I phone, apologizing for being a nuisance, for my not-knowing. They book me in. The appointment, it turns out, is well overdue.

Later, it will become clear that this was not an unusual story for pregnant women during the pandemic. Face-to-face appointments in antenatal care were reduced, with some areas switching to phone calls and video appointments for routine check-ups. Data from eighty-one UK maternity units suggests that the number of screening tests for conditions such as gestational diabetes fell, as did the number of growth scans performed. In some cases, specialist care – such as for pregnant women with epilepsy – was cancelled.[1] Some women reported being told they could not have certain procedures, such as a membrane sweep to help stimulate labour, because it was too much of an infection risk.[2]

On top of this, it emerged that pregnant women sometimes actively avoided seeking help if it meant going into hospital, doing what they believed was best, as per the government messaging at the time: 'Stay Home. Protect the NHS. Save Lives.' This had devastating consequences. As well as contributing to maternal deaths, we now know that there was a sharp spike in the number of stillbirths at the beginning of the pandemic – and not due to Covid-19 itself. After staff noticed an unusually high number of stillborn babies at St George's Hospital in London during the first lockdown, obstetrician Professor Asma Khalil conducted a study to try to find out why. Initially, her team thought it might be down to infection from the virus. However, while it's since been found that Covid-19 infection while pregnant may indeed raise the risk of stillbirth, none of the mothers at St George's whose babies died had had the virus. 'The most likely theory is that because the initial public health message was "Stay at home, don't come to hospital", women didn't come in when they had a problem, such as reduced foetal movements,' Professor Khalil tells me, 'perhaps because they didn't want to overload the system, or they were afraid of catching Covid.' Further research, which Professor Khalil and others published in the *Lancet* in 2021, backs this up, she says, as the number of women attending out-of-hours maternity services dropped by 20 per cent during this stage of the pandemic, compared with the same period in the previous year.[3] What's more, after the Department of Health and Social Care adjusted its messaging, with campaigns urging pregnant people to get any concerns checked out, stillbirth rates returned to expected levels.

Clare Murphy, of the British Pregnancy Advisory Service, suggests to me that one of the key lessons from the pandemic is how pregnant people react to health messages. 'A couple of studies have looked at women's experiences during the pandemic and also how women interpreted risk messages, and both studies independently found that, if anything, women overinterpreted the rules on social distancing,' she tells me. 'It turns on its head this idea that you need to give pregnant women strong warnings. Actually, if you give women a warning, they take it to an absolute extreme.' She continues: 'We would be much better off if we started to think about public-health messaging around pregnancy with that at its foundation: that women are minded to do their very best by their pregnancy. In the pandemic, pregnant women took social distancing to its absolute extreme because they were so concerned.'

We also did it because we are primed to err on the side of extreme caution. A frustrating reality of pregnancy is that when medicine doesn't know what the actual level of risk might be, the answer is almost always: better not. *Better safe than sorry.* After four miscarriages, I am more than used to playing

things 'safe'. No running. No caffeine. Not even a sip of alcohol. No dyeing my hair. No painkillers. But in the first weeks
of lockdown, staying safe takes on a whole new dimension. I
go nowhere, I see no one.

I make it to the third trimester. I pass the twenty-eight-week
mark just as the press briefings and news bulletins start to suggest we have reached the peak of daily infections and deaths
from the virus. The numbers, finally, seem to be coming down.
This is a relief, if only a partial one. At the start of lockdown,
my biggest fear had been that the peak would coincide with
when I went into labour and that hospitals would be overrun.
And yet – there is a suggestion that the final months of pregnancy are when the chance of being seriously ill with the virus
is highest, possibly due to reduced lung capacity as the growing
baby stretches you to your limits. The exact level of risk is still
unclear, with the advice to pregnant people hastily assembled
from individual case studies from the current pandemic, the
effects of other viruses in pregnancy, and from seasonal flu. But
just as I feel more vulnerable to the virus than ever, the conversation is starting to turn towards normal life resuming, with
the prospect of people returning to workplaces and schools.

Dan and I have our routine. He wears gloves to the supermarket. We quarantine any packages that arrive in the porch for
seventy-two hours. We take daily walks where we are unlikely
to pass other people, skirting the fields and sometimes climbing
a modest hill, from where we can look back at the villages
below, the heavy brow of a moorland ridge above us, and the
gleaming towers of the city beyond. Whichever route we pick,
it is increasingly slow and effortful on my part. The lambs make
us smile as we pass, particularly when they are too young to
have learned to be afraid, pressing their curious faces up at us
through the hedgerows.

Ensconced like this, it sometimes feels like the pandemic has brought our experience of pregnancy closer to the curve of normality. For so long, I didn't feel pregnant in the same way as other women. I couldn't trust my body enough for me to be able to do things that others took for granted: the early-bird bookings of antenatal classes, the shopping for baby things, the hospital bags packed long before the due date. Only now, we are experiencing pregnancy as everyone is. Or rather, everyone else is experiencing pregnancy our way. Right now, no one else is having a baby shower or browsing department stores for the perfect pram, either. This is not exactly a reason to be cheerful. There is little joy in seeing the painful parts of miscarriage, trying to conceive, and pregnancy after loss, come alive to others through lockdown living. After a miscarriage, particularly an early miscarriage, your loss exists only to you and perhaps your partner. Even if you tell a few people, there is often little evidence of your pregnancy – no outwardly visible bump, no pictures. Normally, of course, this is exacerbated by the weird codes of secrecy around the first trimester. But now, in lockdown, no one's pregnancy exists in any visible, physical sense to anyone outside their household bubble. The pain of this, the lack of connection other people feel to your pregnancy – your *baby* – and the way you are denied those relationships, is not exactly the same as the pain of pregnancy loss. But if you listen closely enough, you can hear its echoes.

Even among people who aren't pregnant, it increasingly feels like the world is more in tune with our mindset. Friends and family describe to us how the pandemic is making them feel: the uncertainty, the disappointment, the sense of life being on hold – all emotions Dan and I have lived with for years now. Disappointment, in particular, is a feeling that is easy to underestimate until it is a daily companion. The rather straight-laced word we package it up in confers something minor, manageable, and polite. But it is nothing of the sort. To describe a miscarriage or losing a baby as 'disappointing' sounds like classic British understatement. But underneath the hotter emotions of shock, anger, and chest-splitting grief, disappointed is what you are. It didn't happen as you hoped it would. Something was denied. Hope was dashed. And that flat, damp feeling can become hardwired. If you are recurrently disappointed, it gets into your bones. *It probably won't work out. Don't get too excited.*

History suggests that in the shadow of an existential threat on a global scale, like a pandemic or war, we may be more inclined to see pregnancy loss as important. As Dr Rosemary Elliot, a senior lecturer in economic and social history at the University of Glasgow, has pointed out, 'From the Boer War and heightened in the First World War, concerns about fertility decline and infant mortality were shared by the medical profession, political elites and social reformers, with the result that an unprecedented level of medical attention, policy and public health engagement focused on women of reproductive age.'[4] This led to early research efforts into treatments to prevent miscarriage, such as synthetic hormones. Newspaper reports from the 1950s describe potential new tests and treatments for miscarriage in terms such as 'a small beginning to a big problem'.[5]

Might we now see a similar boom in interest in protecting early pregnancy? The Covid-19 pandemic laid bare the extent of many fractures and fault lines in healthcare – from staff shortages to inequality of outcome between people of different backgrounds. Likewise, it exposed holes in our knowledge and the potential hidden costs of such data gaps. For one thing, it revealed just how dangerous our blanket exclusion of pregnant women from medical trials can be – ironically, a convention that has grown from a desire to keep pregnant women and their babies safe. This abundance of caution has not come from nowhere. In the 1950s and 1960s, pregnant women were marketed an over-the-counter drug, thalidomide, for insomnia and morning sickness that they were told was perfectly safe, but which in fact caused babies to be born with shortened limbs, or no limbs at all, as well organ damage and disabilities such as blindness. An estimated half of thalidomide babies died in the months after birth. It has also been suggested that the drug could have contributed to as many as 10,000 stillbirths and miscarriages in the UK, though this may not have been recognized at the time. A similar but lesser-known story is that of diethylstilboestrol, or DES, which was prescribed to prevent miscarriage from the 1940s up until the 1970s. Sometimes referred to as 'silent thalidomide', this synthetic oestrogen was given to women in the mistaken hope it would prevent pregnancy loss. However, it was later found to increase the risk of rare forms of vaginal and cervical cancer in the daughters of women given the drug – in many cases robbing them of their fertility. Both of these stories are still deployed as reminders of what went wrong before we knew the harm that could be done by substances taken in pregnancy. Yet this is an oversimplification, because both medical scandals are not only about what can happen when there isn't sufficient evidence – they are examples of how drug companies and doctors actively *ignored* evidence that did exist. DES continued to be prescribed to millions long after research showed that, not only did the drug not prevent miscarriage, it potentially *increased* the risk of pregnancy loss.[6] And despite researchers establishing the link with cancer in 1971, DES wasn't banned in the US and UK until two years later and continued to be prescribed in parts of Europe as late as 1983. As for thalidomide, its German manufacturers insisted that it had no effect on a developing baby, even though they had neglected to try to establish this in any way. It's a subtle distinction, but an important one – these frightening cautionary tales were not born only out of accidental harm and a lack of long-term study results but out of something far more insidious: neglect and an apparently ingrained disregard for women's physical safety, and that of their babies. Arguably, a similar indifference and abnegation of duty exists in today's reluctance to even attempt to see how medications, treatments, and vaccines might affect pregnancy.

As is the default approach for trials into new drugs and vaccines today, those who were pregnant or breastfeeding were excluded from all of the original vaccine trials for Covid, as well as many trials into possible treatments. But many experts believe this approach is outdated. As a group of UK researchers warned back in August 2020, 'we may face the paradoxical situation of recommending vaccination for a risk group in which the vaccine is untested'.[7] This is exactly what happened. When Covid vaccines were first rolled out, they were not recommended for all pregnant people because there was not yet any data on their safety or efficacy. This advice changed several months later, but the tone was set. Hesitancy reigned, to shattering effect. More pregnant or recently pregnant women in the UK died with Covid-19 in the pandemic's third wave – after vaccines were available – than in the second or first waves. In October 2021, six months after the official advice changed, it was reported that almost a fifth of the most critically ill coronavirus patients in England were pregnant women. It's been estimated that by the same point in time around only 15 per cent of pregnant women* had had both doses of the vaccine required for full protection. There were reports of pregnant or breastfeeding women who *did* choose to get vaccinated being turned away. Sometimes, antenatal clinics and midwives explicitly warned pregnant women against the vaccine on the basis that there was not enough evidence yet. Again and again, we run into this same, old idea: *Better safe than sorry*. If women didn't feel safe to get vaccinated, this is palpably not their fault.

---

* Guess what? The precise figure doesn't exist, as England doesn't keep data linking vaccines with pregnancy and birth. This 15 per cent estimate is based on data from Public Health Scotland.

It is the culture we have created, one which complacently accepts knowledge gaps about pregnant bodies – and, in this case, it cost women their lives.

Vaccine hesitancy not only puts unvaccinated individuals at risk, it ultimately endangers entire populations. And fears and misinformation about what vaccination could do to fertility fuelled this. There were (unfounded) rumours that there had been a sharp rise in the number of miscarriages reported to vaccine-monitoring schemes, for example.[8] It is hard to dispel misinformation spreading through the internet. It is even harder if you don't have the full facts to counter it with – basic facts, like the actual number of miscarriages that happen each year. This is not to say that scientists aren't now clear that Covid vaccines are safe and will not compromise fertility: they are. There is now good evidence that shows vaccination makes no difference to fertility, with clinical trial data showing no differ-ence in unintended pregnancy rates between vaccinated and unvaccinated people, and no difference in pregnancy rates for fertility clinic patients either. Vaccination also does not appear to affect sperm quality, the ability of an embryo to implant, or to increase miscarriage rates. But imagine how much easier put-ting minds at ease might have been if we'd had more granular detail about the complex interplay between the immune sys-tem, vaccinations, the menstrual cycle, and pregnancy, right from the get-go?

The pandemic was a brutal reminder of the importance of expert knowledge and reliable information. The creation of vaccines for a new disease in less than a year also showed us what was possible. Yet this was not a simple parable of what we can achieve if we put our minds to it; we shouldn't make the mistake of assuming that this miracle of science was performed from scratch. Like all apparent overnight successes, the vaccines were years in the making. Scientists had been working on the technology used by the Pfizer vaccine for more than two decades. Likewise, the funding grants that ultimately led to the Oxford–AstraZeneca vaccine have been traced back to at least 2002. Meanwhile, much of the work that paved the way for the record-breaking response to Covid-19 in 2020 came from theoretical preparation for a 'Disease X'. What if a future Disease X was to trigger an epidemic of pregnancy loss? It shouldn't take this admittedly Atwoodian scenario to make us appreciate the significance of what we don't know; of how relatively little medicine has to offer for people who lose pregnancy after pregnancy. After all, writ large, not being able to stay pregnant spells extinction for a species.

In some ways, the scale of loss wrought by a global pandemic makes talking about miscarriage harder than ever. The loss of more than 6 million lives – 6 million friends, lovers, mothers, fathers, siblings and grandparents – dwarfs your personal grief for a person who didn't quite exist yet. And yet, paradoxically, the pandemic may also have made it easier for people to understand both the emotions and the inherent virtue in more research. We are perhaps now uniquely placed to appreciate the value of such knowledge: how what we don't know can suddenly come to matter in ways we cannot yet see.

Right now, though, I cannot guess or even dream that by the end of the year we will have approved the first vaccines against Covid-19. I am still taking pregnancy one heavy day at a time. It is on an otherwise unremarkable weekend morning, a week or so into the third trimester, that I start to worry I cannot feel the baby moving – that I haven't felt them moving in quite a while. Normally, when I wake up, I am greeted by rooting and writhing. But today as I sip my first cup of tea, my stomach is still; becalmed. Breakfast also doesn't stir my usually rowdy tenant. I take a shower. I pace up and down like a caged animal, and still nothing. I do not really want to go to the hospital, not now, not when infections are still so high. But I also do not want to stay at home and risk doing nothing. I phone the maternity unit, who tell me to come in.

'We'd always rather you came in.' The midwife I speak to is calm, but firm. 'Try not to worry, lovely.' She pauses and then says what I know is coming; what I am dreading. 'But I'm afraid you will have to come in alone.'

11

'Women's stuff'

(May 2020 – 30 weeks pregnant)

I'm waiting to find out if the baby's heart is still beating, in a room I've not waited in before. It's tucked away, deep inside the maternity unit. There's no one else here but me. It is hot in the particular way that a sealed room gets hot on a sunny day; the air tightly packed, baked under glass. In my handbag I have a magazine, which I don't read, and my lucky grey jumper. When a midwife walks me through to another room, where they can put me on a machine to monitor the heartbeat, there is another woman in the opposite bay, who, from the sound of what the doctor is telling her, is in the early stages of labour and needs to be admitted. If our baby is found to be struggling, is this what they will do for me? Would they do an emergency caesarean section? An induction? I don't actually know how things could play out from here. I have known for weeks that intervention to save this pregnancy is now, theoretically, possible. But I have not considered the actual mechanics. I haven't got a hospital bag packed yet. More than that, I haven't actually

bought any of the things you are supposed to put in such a bag.
No nappies. No sleepsuits. No cheap nightie to wear during
labour.

The midwife takes two elastic belts out of a polythene
packet: one powder blue, one powder pink. 'These are yours
now – you keep them,' she tells me, the plastic crackling
between her hands. She doesn't add 'for next time', but I force
my brain to hear it that way. There *will* be a next time. There
will be a heartbeat that could theoretically be monitored
another day. *Please.*

The fabric belts are looped around me to hold two round
transducers in place against the bare mound of my stomach.
They connect to a machine which nudges out a sheet of paper,
like a lie-detector test. The midwife explains what each zig-
zagging line means – one is the foetal heart rate, the other will
measure the tension in my abdomen, which, indirectly, suggests whether my uterus is contracting or not. She also gives
me a handheld clicker, which I am to press every time I feel the
baby moving. The baby is still quiet, but there is, at least, a
heartbeat for the machine to trace. I breathe out. I am left
attached to the machine for twenty minutes to see what happens. To see if the lie-detector gives anything away. I text Dan,
who is, once again, waiting outside in the car.

There is a fundamental division of labour in pregnancy:
someone has to do the carrying. Someone's body has to bear
the weight of that new person inside their own. You cannot
take turns, even if you wanted to. This means that, often, in
pregnancy one half of a partnership experiences it as a relative
outsider. An enterprise that is supposed to unite you in new,
profound ways, necessarily splits your perspectives. Right now,
Dan might be literally being kept on the outside, barred from
the hospital by pandemic restrictions, but it is not the first time
that pregnancy has imposed distance between us. If you were
to ask Dan how long it took for us to conceive our first

pregnancy, his answer, I suspect, would be different to mine. The months did not leave such an impression on him. He did not feel the same pressure or imposition on his daily life. As a friend who was trying to conceive around the same time told me, sagely, when I was getting impatient: it feels different when it is not your body. The physical imbalance between mine and Dan's experience of trying for a baby has mostly gone unsaid between us. It is so obvious and insurmountable that there is almost nothing to say about it. Though I know, at times, he has felt guilty.

In four years – aside from completing a form outlining his basic medical history when we were first referred to the recurrent-miscarriage clinic – while I have been scanned, probed, pricked for multiple phials of blood, and put under general anaesthetic twice, Dan has not been required to so much as cough and say 'ah'. The underlying assumption is that miscarriage must always be down to something a woman's body is or isn't doing; how it might be misbehaving, while men and their contribution to the pregnancy are largely left out of the picture. For example, semen is not routinely analysed for recurrent-miscarriage patients. And yet, as Dr Channa Jaya-sena, a consultant in reproductive endocrinology and andrology (male reproductive health) at Imperial College London and Hammersmith Hospital, tells me, 'It's plausible and probable that there must be something about sperm that could go wrong to lead to miscarriage.' After all, a sperm cell contributes 50 per cent of the genetic information required to build a human. In 2019, noting the historical lack of interest in how male biology might contribute to pregnancy loss, Dr Jayasena and a team of researchers at Imperial set up a study to address this, and they found that male partners of women who've had three or more miscarriages tend to have higher levels of damage to their sperm's DNA (sometimes called DNA fragmentation) – twice as high, in fact, compared to the control group of similar men, whose partners had not had miscarriages.[1] It's believed this kind of sperm damage could be down to bacteria-killing chemicals called reactive oxidative species, which are normally a 'tool used by white blood cells to protect against infection', explains Dr Jayasena, who likens the process to 'the way that bleach can damage things'. As well as more DNA damage, the semen samples from men whose partners had recurrent miscarriage were found to have a four-fold increase in the amount of reactive oxidative species compared to the control group. Now, researchers are exploring what might be causing such raised levels of oxidative stress and, in turn, how it might be treated. One likely culprit is undiagnosed infections, which could mean 'sperm are getting damaged, caught in the crossfire, as it were', says Dr Jayasena. 'These infections may not be aggressive – most men may not know they have them; they may not be STIs [sexually transmitted infections]; they may be infections from urine or faeces that infect the prostate, for example. And many of these infections might manifest only as a bit of an ache, or even nothing.'

High levels of body fat may also increase the activity of reactive oxidative species, according to Dr Jayasena. Genetics is also likely to come into play, somehow. 'We know that many diseases have two components,' he explains. 'One is something in the environment or your behaviour that leads to the disease. And the other is a predisposition, something about your make-up. If some men do have this risk of recurrent pregnancy loss, could there be some genetic factors that change their make-up, which makes them more likely to have sperm DNA damage?'

There are still a lot of basics we don't know when it comes to male fertility. 'Fertility and miscarriage are almost unique in medicine, because you have to study two people,' says Allan Pacey, a professor of andrology at the University of Sheffield. 'That makes it harder.' Not least because we have not been studying both sides equally. That men are an afterthought in

miscarriage and infertility is 'one of my bug bears', Dr Ippok-
ratis Sarris tells me. Dr Sarris is a consultant in reproductive
medicine and the director of King's Fertility, a fertility clinic in
London. He suggests to me that, out of all the published papers
on fertility, only around 2 per cent relate to male infertility and
reproductive health. Which, when you consider that an issue
on the male side is found in about half of all cases where a couple cannot conceive, starts to seem not so much an imbalance as
completely unhinged. That the origins of infertility fall in a
roughly even gender split seems so unsurprising it shouldn't
need saying. Yet the idea that fertility is a predominantly female
issue runs deep in our imagination. In fact, 'in about 25 per cent
of cases, infertility is attributable to something on the female
side, and for 25 per cent it's the male side. For another 25 per
cent it's both, and in the final 25 per cent the cause remains
unknown,' Dr Sarris tells me. Low sperm counts are a factor
for about one in three couples who are seen for infertility,
according to the NHS.

Even so, the burden of treatment for infertility is carried almost
exclusively by women. Aside from a couple of surgical procedures
to correct blockages that may be stopping sperm being ejaculated,
there are few treatments for male infertility – at least, not any that
are administered directly to the male body. Instead, low sperm
count, poor motility (the way the sperm move), or abnormal
morphology (their shape) tend to be addressed with something
called intracytoplasmic sperm injection, or ICSI, which means a
single sperm is injected directly into an egg cell, but this also
involves someone's female partner going through IVF, which for
them means daily drug injections for several weeks and undergoing two surgical procedures, one under sedation. The hormone
regimen has side effects ranging from bloating, bruising from
injections, tiredness and hot flushes to a risk of a complication
called ovarian hyperstimulation syndrome (OHSS), which is a
reaction to the drugs that stimulate egg production, causing the

ovaries to become very large and painful, and sometimes to leak
fluid, causing severe swelling. IVF pregnancies are also slightly
more likely to be ectopic than pregnancies conceived naturally. In
short, it's invasive treatment – invasive treatment that many, many
women are incredibly grateful exists, and one that more still wish
would be made available to them; nonetheless it is a far-from-ideal
situation. Especially when it is treating something that has not
gone 'wrong' in their body in the first place. This isn't about blame.
No one is to 'blame' for infertility, male or female. This is about
women's bodies being made to pay for medicine's complacency.
The trade-off might be a just-about-acceptable one if IVF had a
high success rate. But it doesn't. In the UK, the average birth rate
per embryo transferred for all IVF patients is 23 per cent. Even in
the best-case scenario, in people under thirty-five the chance of
success is 31 per cent per transfer. People often have to go through
repeated cycles of medication and embryo transfers to eventually
have a baby. Often, there are no satisfying answers for why a particular cycle hasn't worked.

How many women's bodies are being cudgelled with medication in an attempt to correct something that, ultimately, lies
outside of themselves, beyond their physical capacity to fix? As
American researchers noted in 2020, 'because of our limited
understanding of the male contribution, women endure the
health risks of treatments for a disease that may not be theirs'.[2]
Others have gone further. In 2018, Professor Chris Barratt, head
of the reproductive medicine group at the University of Dundee
and director of the Global Male Reproductive Health Initiative,
wrote that women 'have suffered invasive treatment, on behalf
of male infertility management, with silent dignity in pursuit of
a baby, but in a world in which we claim to be addressing inequalities between men and women, this is a stand-out example
of the infringement of basic human rights and dignity'.[3]

Professor Pacey attributes this absence of male biology, at least
in part, to a lack of specialists in male fertility. 'If you are a woman

and you have a fertility problem, you get referred to a gynaecologist. If you are a man and you have a fertility problem, you get referred to a gynaecologist,' he tells me. 'There is an imbalance there. This is not to say that gynaecologists aren't skilled, but they didn't specialize in gynaecology to then spend their lives looking at men.' And just as miscarriage isn't a sub-specialty that gynaecologists can train in, there isn't a defined route for doctors and scientists to specialize in andrology either. This is true around the world. According to one recent estimate, there are fewer than 200 andrologists in America.[4] Professor Pacey adds: 'You get into circular arguments, which is: what's the point of having a male fertility specialist, because there's nothing that can be done anyway. But if nobody's working in that space, you're not going to move it forwards and find something that *can* be done.'

Not unlike miscarriage, what we don't know about male fertility starts with the very basics: there is no official male fertility rate. 'Believe it or not, we don't even know how common male fertility issues are,' Professor Pacey tells me. 'At a very fundamental level, we're still scrabbling around in the dark.' National fertility rates do not include male biology; instead they are measured as births per 100,000 women. 'This means all of our epidemiological statistical data is based around women, which is understandable, because there's a birth event,' explains Professor Pacey. 'That event is undeniable, people witness it, it usually happens under medical supervision, and so there are relatively few births that happen without somebody knowing.' Paternity – and therefore male fertility – is a different matter, though. While fathers are recorded on birth certificates, this, for all sorts of important social reasons, is not compulsory or definitive. It is also not recorded officially, as a measure of male fertility. Biological paternity, after all, is not the same as being a father. 'A paternity is very difficult to record,' says Professor Pacey. 'In order to answer that fundamental question about how common male fertility is, we'd have to compulsorily DNA-test all fathers to get the data. And that's a step too far; it seems like an intrusion. But until we did something like that, we wouldn't truly understand what the incidence of fertility or infertility was in men.' He continues: 'That then feeds into the narrative about whether male infertility is getting more common or whether sperm counts are declining. Often those two things are seen in parallel, but actually they're not the same.' In other words, even if sperm counts are declining – and there is evidence to suggest that they might be[5] – it is difficult to know the absolute truth of how male fertility is or isn't being compromised by this, in terms of how many babies are being born.

At the other end of the scale, we still know relatively little about the molecular components of sperm; that is, what's going on inside these tiny cells – the smallest of all human cells – and how it might contribute to infertility and miscarriage. The kind of semen analysis done for most fertility patients tends to look at basic external characteristics of sperm such as the quantity, shape, and how they move. But, as researchers pointed out in 2020, this tells you nothing about the internal workings of sperm, including potential defects, which could be a source of unexplained infertility.[6] For example, DNA fragmentation, which could have implications for both miscarriage and the success of IVF treatment, can be found in the sperm of men who have had otherwise positive results from a semen analysis. One small study from 2015 found that men whose partners had previous miscarriages or recurrent rounds of unsuccessful IVF treatment were more likely to have chromosomal errors within their sperm than men whose partners had not; however, their sperm samples often appeared normal.[7]

Could it be that in miscarriage – as in infertility – male biology is just as likely to contribute as a woman's? At the moment, this potential role is barely acknowledged at all. It's well known that being older, being overweight, smoking, or drinking heavily can compromise a man's sperm health (along with other, less obvious, lifestyle factors, such as wearing tight underwear and frequent use of hot tubs or taking hot baths). Yet, these have barely been considered as contributing factors in miscarriage. A systematic review of evidence published in 2021 found a total of just eight studies that looked at the link between a male partner who smokes and pregnancy loss. From this, the researchers concluded that smoking more than ten cigarettes a day *before* conception does indeed increase the risk that someone's partner will miscarry. However, the researchers could identify only five studies that investigated an association with how much alcohol a man drank and were unable to establish a clear link either way. And they found no studies at all that evaluated the difference a male partner's weight made to miscarriage risk.[8] Currently neither the NHS, the American Pregnancy Association, the Royal College of Obstetricians and Gynaecologists, nor Planned Parenthood make any reference in their patient information on miscarriage about the role of sperm or paternal lifestyle.

This is in stark contrast to the way women's lifestyles are scrutinized – how we scrape over our own behaviour, looking for reasons the pregnancy might have ended. Traditionally, women have 'taken the slack – and the blame', Dr Jayasena agrees. Just as due attention hasn't been paid to the role a man's body might play, has medical research into miscarriage been unduly weighted in favour of explanations that implicitly blame women? Studies that look at women's behaviour during pregnancy – how much coffee or alcohol they drink, what they eat, and whether they exercise – certainly generate a disproportionate amount of interest. I won't deny that such studies are inevitably interesting to us when we are in the middle of trying to conceive or reeling from a pregnancy loss. But are we so irresistibly drawn to such studies because they align with a deep-rooted belief that a woman is solely responsible for her pregnancy, and by extension at fault when she miscarries? Are we primed to ask certain kinds of questions – and to accept their answers – because they confirm what we are already made to feel?

Because, when it comes to miscarriage, it's amazing how frequently both the things women worry about and the targets for scientific investigation chime with patriarchal norms and codes for acceptable female behaviour. The things we worry about most are the things that, on some level, we feel we shouldn't be doing. For example, according to gynaecologist and miscarriage specialist Professor Lesley Regan, women who have had a previous termination are often 'full of guilt and remorse that the termination may in some way be the cause of the later miscarriages', or even that it represents 'some form of divine retribution'.[9] But evidence has shown convincingly that a safely performed, uncomplicated abortion does not raise the risk of subsequent miscarriage. 'Unfeminine' exercise such as training with weights, intense workouts, and running also often come up as reasons someone feels they may have triggered their own miscarriage. As does job stress and working long hours. The evidence on these is more nuanced.* But the small differences suggested by some studies seem disproportionate to the amount of worry generated in this area. Continuing to do moderate exercise that you are used to doing does not bring on a miscarriage.† Neither

---

* There is some evidence, for example, that women with a history of miscarriage who did large amounts of high-intensity exercise around the time of conception are more likely to have a very early, pre-clinical pregnancy loss (i.e. a pregnancy that is miscarried around the time someone's period was due) compared with those with lower activity levels, whereas studies in elite female athletes, who train much harder, even in pregnancy, than non-athletes, have found it makes no difference to the risk of miscarriage. Comparing the difference that exercise makes is tricky, because it is easily confounded by pregnancy symptoms – if someone feels able to exercise a lot in the first trimester and miscarries, it might be the lack of symptoms that's significant, indicating something about how their pregnancy is unfolding, rather than the exercise itself.

† Generally, it is accepted that continuing to do exercise that your body is used to does not increase the risk of miscarriage, as long as you do not exercise to exhaustion (if you are too breathless to talk, this suggests it's too strenuous). The only

does a bad week at work or being worried about a presentation. Sex is another example. Many women worry that having sex in early pregnancy might increase their risk of miscarriage, sometimes avoiding it altogether. This is not all in our pretty little heads. As recently as the 1980s, medical textbooks actually listed sex or 'coitus' as a potential cause of miscarriage that should therefore be avoided. Today, most doctors and online health advice reassure you that sex in early pregnancy is fine and emphasize that it will not have been a reason for miscarriage. But – wait for it – no one appears to have actually done a definitive study to find out what difference sex actually makes, if any.[10]

What's more, just as society finds ways to admonish both women who enjoy sex too much *and* women who don't enjoy it enough, so too with miscarriage medicine. In 2019, a group of researchers from the Netherlands conducted a study into the link between recurrent miscarriage and how often women gave blow jobs. *Blow jobs.* 'We hypothesized that women with recurrent miscarriage have had less oral sex compared to women with uneventful pregnancy,' wrote the authors in the *Journal of Reproductive Immunology.* The study involved asking ninety-seven women who were patients at a recurrent-miscarriage clinic, most of whom had had four or more miscarriages, about their sex lives and comparing their answers to those from 137 women who had not had miscarriages. This revealed that only 56.9 per cent of the recurrent-miscarriage patients said they gave their partners blow jobs and swallowed the semen, compared with 72.9 per cent of the women in the control group. Accordingly, the authors concluded that 'this study suggests a possible protective role of oral

---

activities explicitly advised against are those where there's a risk of falling or contact sports. In the past, I'd try to remind myself that if going for a run or a long walk induced pregnancy loss, no woman would ever need an abortion – though I still didn't run in any of my subsequent pregnancies after my first miscarriage.

sex in the occurrence of recurrent miscarriage'.* There are many problems with this study. Not least, when the scientists added in what's known as 'imputted data' – statistical guesses for data that was missing from their original findings – the correlation disappeared. But I don't actually object to the line of enquiry altogether. When it comes to miscarriage research, I'm a pragmatist. Whatever it takes. If the answer is blow jobs, the answer is blow jobs. And the basis for this particular piece of research was to add to understanding about the maternal immune system and to explore whether exposure to immune components in semen, absorbed via the gut, before pregnancy has any impact. There have been many scientific studies that sound silly but which led to serious breakthroughs.

All the same, we have to ask why we privilege certain topics over others, especially when the field of what we don't know is so wide. Also, scientists have a responsibility to consider what assumptions might be underpinning their work – or what assumptions their work might play into. Because, while I'm not saying this was the researchers' motivation, their study was widely, gleefully reported. '*Swallowing a partner's semen could help you have a baby, scientists claim*' declared one headline. One site even saw fit to illustrate their write-up of the study with a stock photo of a woman licking a banana. And it wasn't only excitable tabloid websites. Even well-intentioned articles attempting to debunk the study still managed to trivialize and titillate. '*Does oral sex prevent miscarriage? Don't get excited, guys*' read the headline on a blogpost for the American Council of Science and Health. Because, of course, the prospect of more blow jobs would make

---

* Amazingly, this is not even the first study to look at blow jobs as a miracle cure for recurrent miscarriage – there was one in 2005 that suggested a link, as well as another in 2000 that concluded there was a possible association between swallowing semen and lower risk of pre-eclampsia.

any man feel so much better about all those lost pregnancies and the fact he isn't a father yet.

What does such research and reporting do to our perceptions of miscarriage? What does it do to people who have miscarried? What does it do to your psyche to be reminded repeatedly – and almost exclusively – that miscarriage can be attributable to women's choices and behaviour? After miscarriage and/or infertility, women sometimes go to extraordinary lengths to improve their chances of having a baby: acupuncture, reflexology, fertility massage, crystal healing beds, super-smoothies, ever-more-expensive fertility supplements, at-home hormone testing, at-home gene testing, gluten-free diets, dairy-free diets, ditching certain skincare products, downing Chinese herbal remedies that taste like pond water. Often, we do these things not because we are mindless, misinformed idiots, but because we need to do *something*. This drive does not come from nowhere. In her 1990 polemic *The Beauty Myth*, Naomi Wolf identified the problem of 'beauty work' – the constant arms race of upkeep and maintenance required of women to look a certain way. Beauty work, she argued, was a new attempt to reassert control over women, taking up their time, energy, and power. All the ways we seek to adjust our lifestyles while trying to conceive, then, function in a similar way. It's fertility work: the appointment admin, the shopping for and sourcing of obscure vitamins and ingredients, the scrutinizing of labels, and endless googling, the constant physical monitoring and policing. Just like Wolf's concept of beauty work, it's 'an imperative for women and not for men', one that flows from the same 'old feminine ideology' and a similar 'dark vein of self-hatred, physical obsessions, terror of ageing, and dread of lost control'. If housework is the 'second shift'*, and beauty work is the 'third shift' that Wolf identified,

---

* A phrase coined by the sociologist Arlie Hochschild to describe the additional labour in the form of household chores and childcare that begins when people – but particularly women – return from paid work outside of the home.

then fertility work is yet another side hustle demanded of women – and not their male partners.

Increasing our knowledge – both in terms of scientific research and public understanding – of how men contribute to infertility and miscarriage could do a lot to let women off this particular hook. If we knew more about the role sperm played, we might be more persuadable that it is not simply on us to work harder and harder at getting and staying pregnant. Because a miscarriage might be set in motion before an egg is even fertilized. Before a single sperm even enters the female body. Before it has even left a man's body.

This kind of uncertainty, then, is something to be borne in partnership, shared equally along with the responsibility for the future health of a pregnancy. Because otherwise, making women carry this burden alone can start to do terrible things to relationships. Dr Sarah Bailey, lead nurse for recurrent-miscarriage care at University Hospital Southampton NHS Foundation Trust, tells me she has had women patients say desperate things to her like: 'My husband married me expecting I'd be able to give him children. What if I'm unable to do that?' or 'What if he goes off with someone else? He has every right to do that because this is all my fault.' Sarah responds: 'It clearly isn't, but there's still that guilt.' Even if you do not explicitly fear that your partner will leave you, it is a terrible thing to wonder if they blame you. But it is an equally terrible thing to see someone you love tear themselves apart because they blame themselves. It's just one more shadow that closes in on you, as you wait, not knowing if you'll ever have the baby you both want; one more twilight question you barely dare ask yourself: where does this end? And who will we be when we get there?

Am I enough for you? Are you enough for me?

Both men and women are caught in a double-bind here. Women's bodies have, historically, been overlooked by medicine to the point of neglect. This in itself contributes to the way miscarriage is perceived and treated today. Yet, because reproduction has been seen as a woman's domain, in this specific context men are also neglected and overlooked by medicine. And so miscarriage and infertility continue to be seen as 'women only' issues, which also affects the status granted to them. Women's bodies are blamed and bear the brunt. But, one way or another, we all lose out.

Because men are affected by miscarriage. They suffer too.

Contrary to gender stereotypes, research suggests that men desire children just as much as women.[11] And while not as much work has been done looking at the psychological impact of pregnancy loss on men as there has been in women, studies suggest that they experience a similar intensity of grief.[12] As with their female partners, the extent of men's feelings about miscarriage is not dictated by how far along the pregnancy was. An early miscarriage is no less real for a man. What is clear, from the studies that have been done, is that although the grief – and sometimes stress, depression, and anxiety – experienced by men is similar to how women feel, men deal with these feelings very differently. They are, for example, more likely to use alcohol and drugs as coping mechanisms, according to one evidence review published in 2017. They may also be more likely to bury themselves in work as a distraction. Often, research suggests, they feel that it is their duty to be strong for their partner, who is going through the miscarriage. Adding to this pressure-cooker of expectation and internalized grief is that men's feelings about miscarriage may not be entirely appreciated by the people around them – or they may even be minimized. This has certainly been true for us. Friends who learned to be delicately mindful of how pregnancy announcements, baby showers, and children's birthday parties might be difficult for me did not always extend that same sensitivity to Dan. The idea that other people's children – and the absence of our own – could cause him pain didn't seem to come as naturally to them.

It should be said that while men's feelings about miscarriage have been relatively under-explored, even less is known about the experience of lesbian women and non-binary people whose partners miscarry. One very small study from 2007, involving just ten lesbian couples, suggests that 'social' or non-gestational mothers (the mother who is not carrying the baby), like hetero-sexual fathers, tended to keep their sadness private and try to be 'the strong one',[13] while a slightly larger study from 2010 sug-gested that, in some ways, 'the experience of loss is amplified for lesbian and bisexual women', because conception for them is almost always deliberate, a logistically more complex and drawn-out process. Often, it involves privately funded fertility treatment using donor sperm, which makes it an expensive process, too. The same piece of research also found that around a quarter (26.8 per cent) of lesbian or bisexual women experi-enced some form of prejudice, heterosexism, or homophobia during their medical care after a miscarriage. This ranged from same-sex partners being 'pretty much ignored' to partners being asked to leave during physical exams (this was in Amer-ica) or, in one case, a clinician mistaking a woman's partner for her mother.[14] Similarly, almost nothing is known about how miscarriage affects gay men who are trying to become fathers through surrogacy, though a couple of studies, which did not look at pregnancy loss directly, have suggested that commercial surrogacy clinics do not afford much space for intended par-ents' emotions when their surrogate miscarries (or, indeed, for the feelings of the surrogate).[15]

There has also been vanishingly little research on how partners – either male or female – experience recurrent miscar-riage. In 2020, researchers behind an ongoing trial into men's experience of repeat pregnancy loss noted how they had been unable to find any previous research that looked at the effects on men of more than a single miscarriage.[16] However, obstetri-cian and miscarriage researcher Professor Siobhan Quenby tells me how questionnaire scores from her recurrent-miscarriage clinic suggest that men can experience just as much anxiety as women. 'It does affect them far worse than we realized,' she says. Men attending recurrent-miscarriage clinics can also exhibit physical signs of enormous stress. Professor Quenby describes to me how her clinic began taking basic health information from male partners, including taking their blood pressure on arrival. 'And when we first started, we were absolutely horrified because we found all these men who were hypertensive [i.e. they had high blood pressure]. So, then we were sending them back to their GP to get their blood pressure checked.' However, she says, those men would then go to their GP and their blood pressure would be fine. 'We realized it wasn't a blood-pressure issue – it's that they're under enormous stress. It really shook us, because we hadn't realized that they're the ones with more physical signs of stress. We had completely underestimated it.' Professor Quenby adds: 'We're really careful now about sitting them down and having a little bit of a chat before we take their blood pressure.'

It does men who are going through pregnancy loss a disservice not to investigate them thoroughly, too – this is something to which men are very receptive, in Dr Jayasena's experience. 'When we did our DNA damage study and we told the men whose partners had recurrent pregnancy loss that they had the problems with their sperm, we were worried, because we thought it may be upsetting and might cause them to feel guilty,' he tells me. 'But for many of them it was actually quite the opposite. Many of them said, "Thank you: thank you for telling me that there's something, for giving me an answer." They liked knowing, they wanted to know, and they felt more involved as a result.' And yet too often in both miscarriage and fertility clinics 'men are ignored', he says. 'They're almost treated like an accessory – as though they're just there to provide the sperm and that's it.'

The reality is men *do* worry that they might be in some way culpable for miscarriage. Underneath all of the cultural messaging that says it must be a fault on the woman's side, that fear remains for men – largely unarticulated. Cam went through a miscarriage with his on–off girlfriend a few years ago, after an unplanned pregnancy. When he found out she was pregnant, he assumed they would get married; instead, they ended up breaking up not long after the loss. A year later, his ex messaged him to say she was expecting a baby with her new boyfriend. 'I couldn't help but think that it meant the miscarriage was my fault: like, fuck, is it me there's something wrong with?' he tells me. 'Here she was having another man's baby, so clearly everything on her end was functioning properly. I know rationally that's not how it works. I know miscarriages are really common. I know that it's nobody's fault. I know the science. But sometimes I can't help worrying that it means I'm going to find it difficult to have children when I eventually meet the right person.'

Acknowledging men in miscarriage is a radical act. Radical, because acknowledging men's emotional response goes against stoic, silent, hypermasculine stereotypes. Radical, because examining male biology in this context confronts ideas about virility. Radical, because it implicates men as equally responsible for life before birth. In short, it challenges some of the oldest, most intransigent ideals in our culture: what it means to be a man, a father.

Indeed, Professor Allan Pacey believes that one of the reasons medical knowledge of male fertility has lagged behind is because as a subject area it lacks a campaigning voice from male patients. Unlike female fertility patients, who he notes are keen to share and trade experiences with other women in a similar position, to contribute to workshops and research efforts, Professor Pacey tells me it can be difficult to get men to discuss infertility. When he gives talks and workshops, he says often the only time men will ask him their questions is by sidling up to him afterwards, while he's queueing for a sandwich. 'I've even had conversations at the urinals,' he adds. It's a reluctance that is easy to overlook. Celebrities talking about IVF treatment and fertility struggles is increasingly common – and yet it is comparatively rare for it to be explicitly stated when there is an issue on the male side. Likewise, studies suggest that half of men going through fertility treatment never talk to anyone about it other than their partner.[17] Ultimately, though, this lack of male perspective and voice 'will be a real Achilles heel in terms of how we push the conversation forward, how we interest politicians, how we attract the next generation of researchers', Professor Pacey concludes.

Both our past and present are full of examples of how areas of healthcare suffer when the only constituents are women. It seems obvious to me that miscarriage as a subject has suffered until now precisely because it has – incorrectly – been interpreted as a female concern alone: 'women's stuff'. Indeed, one researcher suggests to me that there was a notable uptick in attention and funding after charities made a concerted effort to include male partners in their awareness campaigns, describing it as a 'master stroke'. 'By getting the partner involved, and by acknowledging their experience, suddenly it doubled the number of people involved,' the researcher tells me. 'It's very clever because now it's everybody's issue.'

Of course, it always was everybody's issue.

Even when attention is paid to miscarriage, it is almost always in a certain social context – one that is seen as domestic, feminized, and niche. Miscarriage is the stuff of women's magazines, Instagram, Mumsnet. It is rarely discussed in a political context outside of women's health. The trivialization of it runs deep. I have lost count of the number of times people have suggested to me that, when it comes to conception, fertility, and pregnancy loss, 'perhaps some things are just unknowable'. Yet we accept the inherent value and attainability of much more outlandish quests for knowledge: exploring other planets, penetrating further and further into the unknown of space. No one tells Elon Musk or Richard Branson that some things might be 'best left alone' (although maybe we should).

I have internalized this, too. I often catch myself questioning to what extent I can reasonably expect and demand progress in this particular area of medicine, when there are so many other sources of human suffering that also want for knowledge and research. Though surely, medicine aside, the origins of human life should be an enticing enough topic for us to take miscarriage more seriously? Sometimes, in the years that I have tried and failed to carry a baby to term, it has felt to me that we know and care more about the beginnings of the universe, tens of billions of years ago, than we do our own embryonic beginnings. Perhaps it seems histrionic to draw such a comparison: the Big Bang versus my miscarriages. And yet, fundamentally, both are mysteries of how we came into existence. So why is one seen as an unimpeachably important line of scientific enquiry, a Big Idea that should matter to all people, both profound and transcendent in its implications, while the other is merely a sad story more commonly confined to the health pages of a women's mag? (As if subjects that matter to women couldn't possibly have universal significance.)

Imperial College London's Professor Phillip Bennett believes that, historically, this relative lack of gravitas has affected not just the availability of funding for work in early pregnancy, but also the calibre of scientists the field attracts. 'It's important to bring really talented scientists into this area and to see the importance of it,' he says. 'I think that is happening now: we're gradually realizing that.' Dr Jayasena agrees. 'It links into all kinds of big questions,' he tells me. Like climate change and the environment, for example. An increased risk of miscarriage has been linked to air pollution, Professor Quenby tells me, while in Bangladesh, rising miscarriage rates have been attributed to rising sea levels, possibly because this has led to women ingesting very high levels of salt, as seawater contaminates freshwater.[18] Meanwhile, some male fertility problems (although not all) could potentially be an early warning sign for future health problems, such as heart attacks and strokes, suggests Dr Jayasena. 'This is still a hypothesis,' he says. 'But one day, I think we will join the dots and realize that, in many cases, male fertility problems are one facet of ill health.' Professor Bennett adds: 'Researchers are realizing now that what happens in pregnancy is important for you when you're an adult. What begins in the womb lasts for a lifetime. And what we are now appreciating is that what happens in pregnancy has a lot to do with what happens around the time of conception and in the first trimester of pregnancy. So, increasingly, focus is on optimizing pregnancy from the very, very start.'

After twenty minutes on the monitor, the midwife reassures me that both traces look fine. The baby's heart is ticking away normally – though, as I still haven't really felt them moving, she sends me for a scan just to be on the safe side. Of course, the minute I sit back down in the waiting room, the baby begins somersaulting inside me, twisting, tucking, and piking, as if with renewed energy. I tell the midwife, who laughs.

'Always the way,' she says, with a smile. At least, I assume from her eyes that she is smiling. Her mouth is obscured by a mask.

The scan is fine. The baby wriggles and covers their face coyly with their hands.

I head back out to the car, where Dan is waiting. My sandals – the only thing that fit comfortably on my feet these days – slap against the hot tarmac of the car park. As I approach, I see my husband, eyes downcast, face affectless, lost in his phone. Sweating and exhausted, for a split second I am jealous that he is the one in the car. I am jealous that this is the way he gets to become a parent, that it has not been him inside, prone and probed, waiting for his body to perform in a particular way. At the same time, I feel profoundly sorry that he cannot know what this is like on the inside: now in more ways than one. It wasn't supposed to be like this. I'd always imagined that, should we make it to this point, this would be when we started to experience pregnancy in a less complicated way – in a way that brought us closer together, when for so long its absence has threatened to make us unreachable to each other. And he has been held at bay from fatherhood for so long. We should be out in the world, as a couple. Me visibly pregnant, him visibly a father-to-be; our experience of this thing we're doing as unanimous as it is possible to get. Instead, here he is, waiting for me – and for his baby – behind glass.

12

'Just stay positive'

(June 2020 – 35 weeks pregnant)

Everywhere Dan and I go, we see rainbows. They appear in bedroom windows and shopfronts. They are sellotaped to conservatories, they are chalked on to pavements and playgrounds, and collaged along hospital corridors. Although it has become a collective symbol for optimism in the face of a global pandemic, a rainbow is also the chosen signifier for a baby born after a previous loss, be it stillbirth, miscarriage, SIDS, neonatal death, or termination for medical reasons. A 'rainbow baby' is the label many now use. So, for us, every child's drawing or home-spun window display has a double meaning. Now, there is a reminder on every street, around every corner, of how close we are getting to having our own 'rainbow' baby. Sometimes this feels like the world is cheering us on. At other points, the symbolism begins to feel oppressive. It is hard enough as it is to think about anything other than my pregnant body and whether I might actually get to bring this baby home. It's an uneasy mix. Just like my feelings about the term 'rainbow baby' in the first place. I like that the term exists; that we've found a way to fill a gap in our vocabulary and acknowledge this experience verbally. I also like the suggestion of sunshine after rain; hope after the storm. Still, sometimes it feels so cutesy it sets my teeth on edge. A kindergarten flattening of a complicated thing.

I thought it would feel easier by now. In fact, as I reach thirty-four weeks, the days start to slow and stretch themselves out to impossible lengths, just like they did in the first trimester. At thirty-four weeks, should a baby arrive, they have the same survival chances as a baby born on their estimated due date – although anything before thirty-seven weeks is still considered premature. More than ever, I feel that, should the baby die, it will be my fault. Unlike in earlier pregnancy, there is no basic developmental reason why they should not live now. Unlike in my other pregnancies, there should be lots doctors can do to help. And the pressure I feel not to miss something – some subtle symptom, some warning sign – is intense. On top of this, two weeks ago, measurements taken at a routine scan suggested that the baby's growth might be slowing down. So now I am having weekly scans to monitor the situation. I struggle to sleep. I wake at odd hours in the night, my mind a coiled spring. It is increasingly hard to concentrate on work, not to mention logistically more difficult to juggle deadlines around the extra appointments, which can take hours. At thirty-five weeks, after another unscheduled weekend trip to the maternity unit to check on the baby's movements, my mum suggests I start my maternity leave early.

'It's time to stop,' she says, in a way that leaves no room to argue.

I am secretly relieved. I had been thinking about stopping, too, but felt it would be a sign of weakness, somehow. There is, after all, ostensibly nothing wrong with me or the baby. The latest growth scan showed improvement. The doctors are no

longer talking about having to deliver the baby early. There is
no physical reason I can't work. And yet there is less and less
space alongside my anxiety for anything else. I have little
energy for anything other than the continuing project of staying pregnant and preparing for a baby I still daren't imagine in
any kind of fine detail. But I am also too far along now to continue doing nothing, especially as most shops are still shut
under lockdown rules. The tempting option of waiting and
buying everything in one department-store sweep, once there
is definitely a baby to buy for, doesn't seem like one we can rely
on. Instead, Dan and I try to save the biggest jobs for the
twenty-four hours immediately after a scan, when we stand the
best chance of feeling relaxed. We have chosen a pram, a car
seat, and a Moses basket this way. Even so, every item and task
is a negotiation. If we're not comfortable decorating a nursery
yet, should we at least get the room painted? I try to reason
with myself that denying ourselves the enjoyment of choosing
things now will not protect us should something happen later.
Sometimes this works; sometimes it doesn't. On the whole, I
defer to Dan and what he feels ready for, because what we don't
say, but both know, is that he will be the one who will have to
pack away any items should they prove surplus to requirements.
The image of my husband quietly taking apart an unused cot in
an empty house is one I fight hard to push from my mind. In
fact, it is only getting clearer and more life-like with every
passing day.

   'It's called the imminence effect,' the health psychologist
Professor Jacky Boivin tells me. 'As we approach something
meaningful – that marks something – and where there could
be threatening information provided, our anxiety levels go
up,' she says. By contrast, when the thing we fear actually
comes to pass, anxiety tends to go down. This is a common
'emotional signature' in medical waiting periods, Professor
Boivin explains. And it seems I am as fearful waiting for

impending labour as I was waiting for those very first scans at the recurrent-miscarriage clinic.

Professor Boivin is one of several researchers behind attempts to develop psychological coping tools that can be used in pregnancy after miscarriage to help with the fear, anxiety, and hypervigilance that can be common companions. What they've come up with is a self-help card of ten statements designed to encourage women to think about positive aspects alongside negative aspects of the situation. The idea is the card is read as a prompt every day, as often as people feel they need it. It uses an established psychological coping technique called positive reappraisal. Statements include things such as: 'During this experience I will find something good in what is happening' or 'Focus on what is important in life' and 'Try to do something meaningful'. 'For example, it can make someone realize how supportive their partner is,' says Professor Boivin. 'Or it makes them realize how strong they are, or makes them notice flowers in their garden,' she adds. 'Being joyful in that particular moment of pregnancy could also be part of it, but that's often very difficult for people because they think being joyful about the pregnancy is going to jinx things.'

This method sounds relatively simple, but it's rooted in both established psychological theory and published research. A positive reappraisal card like this was first tested for people who were pregnant after miscarriage by Dutch researcher Henrietta Ockhuijsen in 2013.[1] Then, in 2020, Dr Sarah Bailey, lead nurse for recurrent-miscarriage care at University Hospital Southampton NHS Foundation Trust, published the results of a larger study in recurrent-miscarriage patients.[2] This was what was known as a feasibility study, intended to prove that a larger, randomized controlled trial was both possible and acceptable to potential participants. While this feasibility study was not designed to calculate exactly how much the coping card could help, 'with the limited statistics that we had, the anxiety levels in the group that used it were less', Sarah Bailey tells me. 'We can't take those figures as evidence, but they were really encouraging to us,' she adds. Bailey, who offers the card to her own patients, is now working on setting up a further trial to show just how beneficial the card could be, in the hope it could be distributed more widely to people who are pregnant after recurrent miscarriage.

Crucially, positive reappraisal is not the same as encouraging people to 'just stay positive'. People are quick to say this sort of thing to you after a miscarriage or when you are pregnant again, without fully appreciating that when you next feel sad and scared, or ruminate on the things that you know can go wrong, you can too easily slide into feeling like you are failing – or that you will be doomed by your own 'negativity'. The point of positive reappraisal – looking for the good that sits alongside the bad – is not to make you more optimistic or downplay the worry you feel at the possibility of a particular outcome (in this case the loss of another baby); the point is simply to help you cope for the time being. It does this by offering a break from the entirely understandable stress and negative emotions you are experiencing, given the situation, explains Professor Boivin. 'It will be very difficult to stop someone from feeling anxious, nervous, and worried,' she says. 'What you need to do is provide them with psychological respite – and that's what this does. It just gives someone a break. It gives them the ability to carry on.'

This is not the same as trying to force yourself to believe that this time it really will work out. It's an important distinction, because the pressure to have *only* positive thoughts is a pervasive kind of magical thinking in pregnancy, especially after infertility and pregnancy loss. And for every person who prescribes daily positive affirmations, there is another who will tell you that it will happen when you stop thinking about it so much: *It'll happen when you stop trying . . . Just go on holiday . . . You know, my sister's friend only got pregnant after she gave up on IVF.* These two schools of thought may contradict each other, but they come from the same basic idea: that the mind of a pregnant person can directly influence what happens in the body. This may have new and shiny incarnations, fuelled by the wellness industry, social media, and disciples of 'manifestation' or the so-called 'Law of Attraction', but it draws from an ancient well of superstition – and not a little sexism. Right through until the eighteenth century (at least), the idea that a mother's thoughts, feelings, and cravings could leave a physical mark on her baby, in the form of birth marks or deformities, was a popular one among the general public. Even doctors and midwives, who didn't believe in such a literal effect, warned against strong emotions and any situation that might elicit these in pregnancy, due to a possible risk of miscarriage or stillbirth. Medical textbooks from the eighteenth century advised women against crowds, losing their temper, hearing distressing stories, and reading sentimental tales, for example.[3] In the post-Freudian 1950s, some doctors and psychiatrists believed that recurrent miscarriage had psychological causes, occurring in women who were anxious about motherhood or doubted their ability to carry a child.[4] Even in the twenty-first century, versions of these kinds of folkloric beliefs persist. One modern study found that 35 per cent of attendees at an antenatal clinic in the US believed pregnant women should avoid upsetting things such as violent TV shows or funerals, according to a 2017 evidence review.[5]

Today, the most common concern about how our thoughts could affect our fertility is through stress. The idea that psychological stress can directly cause a miscarriage is a pernicious one – and a myth, according to Professor Boivin. 'Whenever I give talks on stress and fertility, there's always somebody with a history of miscarriage who comes at the end and thanks me for reassuring them that they did not cause their miscarriage,' she tells me. Stress is complicated. Clearly, mental health is not irrelevant when it comes to our physical health and doctors increasingly appreciate how the two are deeply entwined. Finding ways to cope in stressful situations – including pregnancy after previous loss – is undeniably important for our well-being. And yet, the notion that stress itself can be a reason for miscarriage, infertility, or fertility-treatment failure comes from a 'misplaced understanding of the interaction between stress and reproduction', Professor Boivin tells me. It's often said that during intense times of stress, the body can shut down some immediately non-essential functions, including reproduction. But this is an oversimplification. 'The other part of that story is that humans have evolved a set of mechanisms to override this,' explains Professor Boivin. After all, reproduction might be 'non-essential' in a short-term sense, but in the long term, it's our *most* essential function. 'The brain can compensate, producing more reproductive hormones, for example, or the reproductive organs stop reacting to the stress hormones. For most people there's no way stress would make a difference,' she says. 'And especially in a context like IVF – when they give you so many drugs to control the process – your level of stress just wouldn't exist as a factor.'

'You can still manage your stress,' she adds. 'Do your relaxation and mindfulness if it helps you feel good. But do it for your quality of life, not because you think the outcome is going to change.'

There *is* disconcerting research that shows a link between miscarriage and stress, however. 'But there's a mistake in that relationship,' argues Professor Boivin. She says studies are often complicated by not adequately accounting for pregnancy history and the stress caused *by* miscarriage in the first place. The two things often co-exist, but it can be hard to unpick which came first. What's more, stressful life events may have an indirect effect on miscarriage and fertility, 'because when people are stressed, they may use different kinds of coping strategies', explains Professor Boivin. 'And those could be things that *do* have a direct impact, such as smoking or drinking or having sex less often, so there's less opportunity to get pregnant.' But this is not the same as stress *causing* miscarriage and infertility. Even so, 'people have a very strong belief about the role of stress and reproductive functioning', says Professor Boivin, 'because stress is something they can control, whereas miscarriage is not.'

Ironically, this can become a source of stress in itself.

I feel guilty all the time that I am not enjoying my pregnancy more. I also worry that how worried I am could be harming the baby. It doesn't matter how much evidence I try to shore myself up with. What I know rationally and what I feel inside slide past each other, without impact, without friction. They are two completely disconnected planes. Recurrent miscarriage is often a medical condition without reason – and perhaps this is why you find yourself existing in a state beyond reason, too. I am superstitious now in a way I never was before. I salute every solitary magpie. I continue to take my lucky grey jumper to hospital appointments even though now, in midsummer, it is definitely too hot to actually wear it.

For me, right now, everything feels like a jinx. I don't want to hope too much, but I fear what being too negative might mean. Buying too much for the baby feels like a jinx, but buying too little doesn't feel particularly auspicious either. Meanwhile, other people's pregnancy announcements and scan photos continue to unsettle me. I still get the same pangs of jealousy I felt when I was immediately post-miscarriage and seemed to see bumps and babies wherever I went. Only now I have no logical reason to be jealous. Perhaps there is never a logical reason to be jealous of someone else's pregnancy: after all, their being pregnant or having a healthy baby does not have any bearing on your chances of doing the same. And yet somehow, on some lizard-brain level, other people's pregnancies feel like a direct existential threat to mine. 'There's an element of magical thinking there – that because *they* are, it won't happen to *me*,' reflects Ana Nikčević, a professor of psychology and mental health at Kingston University and practitioner psychologist, whose research has looked at women's needs after pregnancy loss. 'I wonder whether, sometimes, we think that way because, in a magical way, we want to protect ourselves from the disappointment. If we give free rein to think "It will happen", then you think you risk being disappointed.'

Sometimes, the detachment from reason that follows a miscarriage verges on delusional. For days, sometimes weeks, after mine, I'd exist in an alternate kind of reality. I'd catch myself believing I was still pregnant, despite all evidence to the contrary. It goes beyond wishful thinking. It's not that I was willing myself to be pregnant again. It went beyond simply wanting it; I genuinely believed I *was* pregnant, still, if only for a few seconds. It would start in the mornings. For a moment, suspended in that place between asleep and fully awake, I wouldn't have remembered, and, briefly, I'd be happy. Then, every time the phone rang, for a fraction of a second I'd think it was the hospital calling to tell me there had been a mistake, a mix-up. They had just got the results: I was, in fact, still pregnant.

Or Dan would say casually, over dinner, 'That reminds me, do you want to hear some good news?' and my brain would snap immediately – implausibly – to: *He's going to tell me I'm pregnant*.

It's the shock, I'd remind myself, when I noticed my own madness. The grief, the trauma. It is disbelief, taken to its literal extreme. It's the same uncanny feeling we get after a bereavement that the deceased could walk through the front door any minute and sit in their favourite chair as if nothing had happened. It's the same bargaining impulse that makes it hard to delete someone's number from our phone when they die, because then it would mean we wouldn't be able to call them. Because then they would really be gone. Because perhaps we can make them stay.

This inability to accept reality seems logical to me – inevitable, even – when there is no explanation for what has happened. The human brain naturally wants to problem-solve, to make meaning from chaos, yet all around you people are telling you there is no meaning: no reason. It makes sense that you would behave unreasonably, too. But being unable to rationalize and process what has happened to us can have darker consequences than a fantastical flicker of hope every time the phone rings.

In 2020, Imperial College London researchers established something seismic. They published a study that concluded almost one in five women who'd had a miscarriage or an ectopic pregnancy met the diagnostic criteria for post-traumatic stress disorder (PTSD). This was true at least nine months after the event (it may be longer, but nine months post-loss was the last point at which researchers surveyed the women). Women in the study experienced enduring intrusive thoughts about their miscarriage, as well as nightmares or flashbacks. Moderate to severe anxiety and depression were also commonplace.

It is certainly an arresting claim. After all, in popular imagination PTSD is something that afflicts war veterans and people caught up in terrorist attacks, not pregnant or recently pregnant women in affluent countries with free, evidence-based healthcare. It's often written that the first cases of what we now call PTSD occurred in men sent to fight in the trenches in the First World War, who then suffered from 'shell shock'. What we would now recognize as PTSD has also been referred to as 'soldier's heart', 'war neurosis', and 'combat hysteria', at various points in history. And perhaps it is this history, along with the fact that the official, modern diagnosis of PTSD in 1980 came about in the aftermath of the Vietnam War, that links this psychological condition so innately with war in our perceptions. Actually, this narrow idea of trauma and subsequent PTSD is unhelpful, according to Dr Claudia Herbert, a consultant clinical psychologist, trauma specialist and author of the book

Overcoming Traumatic Stress. Instead, it's generally accepted that PTSD can follow a range of experiences: being mugged, sexual abuse, a car accident, a bereavement, childbirth – and, yes, miscarriage.

'Psychologically speaking, a trauma is any event that at the time was overwhelming and the person it happened to didn't have the inner or outer resources to deal with it,' Dr Herbert tells me. 'It can be anything that is so overwhelming that it potentially triggers our autonomic nervous system to go into a survival response.' The autonomic nervous system is a largely unconscious bodily system that governs functions such as heart rate and breathing – things we do without needing to think about it, because they are far too important and it would be far too inefficient to rely on our conscious brain to do them (not least because of our pesky habit of going to sleep at night). In times of stress, parts of this system can be activated to take over for us – sometimes called the 'fight or flight' response. 'It's a system that takes us out of directly conscious action,' says Dr Herbert. 'It's an older system within us, controlled by the reptilian centre of our brain, that takes over in situations where, if we only acted through our conscious brain, our reactions would be perceived as being too slow to keep us safe. The unconscious brain takes over, because the situation – whatever it is – in that moment takes us to the boundaries of acceptable danger and is registered as a threat to survival.' Crucially, in terms of miscarriage, she says, 'that can be our own survival, or it could be the survival of somebody we feel we're responsible for – including a baby we may have only recently started to bond with'.*

This activation of the autonomic nervous system primes us to respond to threatening situations. Our heart beats faster to

---

* A separate 2020 study found that some partners of women who miscarry also experience PTSD-like symptoms in the month following the loss.

pump more blood to our muscles and organs, our muscles engage, hormones such as adrenaline surge through us so we can run faster, move more explosively, think faster. 'But at the same time, these unconscious responses prevent our conscious brain from processing what's happening to us properly, in the way it would normally work through something during non-threatening situations,' explains Dr Herbert. Essentially, as this subconscious system takes over, the memories of that moment get stuck. And the flashbacks, nightmares and other encroaching symptoms are the mind and body's attempts to work it through after the event. 'It's your body reminding you that there's something there you haven't fully processed, if you like,' says Dr Herbert. 'Equally, another reaction to trauma is to withdraw. We might shut down emotionally, because it feels safer not to share what has happened. There can also be symptoms of depression; often this is diagnosed without realizing that trauma is at the root of it.' It can also manifest as problems in relationships, anxiety, anger and trouble sleeping – all noted as common after-effects of miscarriage by the Imperial researchers.

And yet, Dr Herbert tells me, 'it isn't inevitable that a miscarriage will be experienced as a full-blown trauma. Although it is very likely that it will always be upsetting – as it's painful emotionally, it's painful physically – it becomes a trauma if there are enough factors coming together to make it so overwhelming in the moment that it's really hard for the brain to work through it and to come to terms with it.'*

According to Dr Herbert, 'Vulnerability factors include the way things are handled in hospital – whether it's explained properly; whether someone is treated in a very cold, procedural way while they are experiencing profound loss for someone

---

* This includes the extent of the physical violence of the miscarriage, although this is also neither definitive nor predictive.

they had already started loving; what medical procedures have had to happen; the severity and amount of physical pain; the way someone's partner or other family members behave at the time; how far along in the pregnancy the loss is happening; whether this is the first child or there are already others; whether there have been any previous losses. There could be a wide number of factors interplaying and what matters is when and how these factors combine so as to potentially feel too overwhelming for an individual.'

There's one more potentially integral piece of the puzzle: how much you know about miscarriage in the first place. I ask Dr Herbert if she thinks a trauma response is made more likely by a lack of prior knowledge of what a miscarriage can be like. 'Absolutely,' she says. Trauma is what happens when we don't feel safe or in control. It seems obvious that the chances of feeling this way increase when you know or understand little about what is happening or what might happen to you in the future. A definition that is sometimes used for trauma is something that is 'outside the range of usual human experience'. A miscarriage, of course, is a sadly all-too-normal part of the human experience − certainly compared with your chances of being caught up in, say, a natural disaster, a terror attack, or a violent car crash. Could it be that the limits we put on conversations around miscarriage are instrumental here? Is it our silences and narrative economies that amplify this experience into something that feels outside our range, way beyond our danger threshold? This is why there's a potential vicious circle here, too, given that one response to trauma is withdrawal: from the memory itself and also from other people. With no frame of reference for what a miscarriage might look like, feel like, hurt like, we are priming women to experience it as a serious trauma. And being traumatized makes it less likely we will talk about it. And so the cycle continues.

To me, this all points in the same direction: how much of the psychological burden could we alleviate if only we knew more about miscarriage? This is why it's so important to hear about it.

I've started having dreams of a kind I have not had since just after my first miscarriage. I'll be walking down the street, or at my desk, or out with friends, and I'll suddenly remember that I've given birth to a baby – a baby I've left at home, alone. In the dream, I race back and search the house frantically, knowing the baby will be dead, that it's been too long, that I've left it unattended for weeks. Night after night, I find these forgotten babies. I find them under my bed, inside drawers, or in carrier bags. It was exactly the same in those raw weeks, four years ago.

It took me a long time to acknowledge that, by any standard, having multiple miscarriages registered as a traumatic experience. Or, at the very least, a significant upheaval. I'd had three miscarriages in the space of nine months before I saw the psychologist who put it to me that perhaps it had been a lot to go through; that perhaps the problem wasn't me and what I saw as my failure to cope. But throughout that first year of trying to have a baby, I'd resisted this interpretation. As much as I recognized what I felt as grief, shock, disappointment and, sometimes, depression, I just felt that I should be managing it better. Hadn't I been told that lots of people go through this? The situation was normal, relatively speaking. It must, therefore, be me who was not.

It was the test results that broke me. Finding out that there was no medical problem after all, and therefore no solution going forward, was what did it. Not straight away. But slowly the days got greyer, fogging into one featureless expanse. I changed departments twice at the newspaper where I worked, but never felt like I was doing a very good job at anything. I stopped drinking alcohol to help with the anxiety. I went to the gym more. I stayed in more. Nothing felt exciting. Nothing felt fun. Some mornings, as I waited to change Tube lines and a train rattled towards the platform, brakes squealing, I'd take an exaggerated step back to be closer to the wall. In that moment, an awareness of what the force of that metal could do to my body consumed me. I vibrated with it and it scared me. But this wasn't a suicidal thought, I told myself. It was the opposite. Wasn't it? Just like when I'd walk past the spiked railings in front of townhouses and think of how those spears could run a person through. That wasn't a suicidal thought, either.

'I think you're depressed,' Dan said, one weekend in February. Or maybe it just felt like it was February – cold and flat.

'I think so too,' I agreed. It had been a relief to have him say it first.

I saw a local counsellor on the NHS. She worked for a small charity, one of a number that help to plug the gaps in psychological services up and down the country. She specialized in pregnancy-related issues. When I spoke to her on the phone, she explained that to get to her therapy room, you had to enter through a shop run by the charity. What she didn't say was that the shop sold second-hand baby gear. As I followed the counsellor past a row of empty cots to get to her office, I tried my best not to cry. This, then, was not going to be the place where I got what I needed. I don't know what was worse – being walked past the bric-a-brac from a life I desperately wanted, or the fact that it hadn't occurred to anybody else that this arrangement might be less than ideal. After that, a doctor friend recommended I look for a clinical psychologist – and pay privately – instead.

Most women who miscarry show symptoms immediately afterwards that are indistinguishable from depression, research suggests.[6] At least 20 per cent meet the clinical diagnostic criteria for anxiety three months later,[7] while some studies have estimated that as many as one in four women are clinically depressed a year on. One piece of research from 2010 suggested that for around one in ten (11 per cent) anxiety or depression does not actually set in until between three and six months later,[8] long after any GP or early-pregnancy unit is going to check in on you (if they do at all). The mental health consequences of miscarriage are serious and prevalent. This has been shown in women all over the world – from China to Mexico, London to Nairobi. I knew this. I'd written articles about it. And yet still I was reluctant to recognize it in myself. I was embarrassed to admit that my mental health was suffering because I so badly wanted a baby. It felt weak, unfeminist even, that my need to carry a child was pushing me to the brink of my sanity. There was something that felt humiliatingly retrograde about it. In some ways, the psychological challenge of miscarriage has become harder, not easier, reflects Professor Nikčević. 'For many women, having children is pertinent to who they are and the meaning of life – not in totality, but as an aspect of a meaningful life,' she says. 'Yet, as we have moved into different spaces as women, it's almost become embarrassing to acknowledge it – as if we will be seen as a woman from the 1950s.'

The idea that an unused womb sends women mad is a particularly unhelpful and rancid strain of misogyny. 'The womb is an animal that longs to generate children,' Plato wrote in 360BC. 'When it remains barren for too long after puberty it is distressed and sorely disturbed, and straying about in the body ... brings the sufferer into the extremest anguish and provokes all manner of disease besides.' This is the theory of hysteria: that an unfulfilled, 'wandering' womb is the source of female illness, both physical and mental. While it may not have been believed in a literal sense for centuries, the catch-all diagnosis of 'hysteria' wasn't completely expunged from medical and psychological textbooks until 1980. And the trope of the infertile or childless woman made crazed, pathetic, or dangerous by her own baby-hunger has never really gone away. Miscarriages, stillbirths, and dead babies hide in trauma plots everywhere, from bestselling beach reads to bingeable TV boxsets. In pop culture, women with my kind of history often end up psychotic, murderous, or tragic baby-snatchers. Against such a backdrop, is it really such a mystery that there's reluctance to acknowledge just how deeply pregnancy loss is affecting you? How it continues to affect you?

Now, with my due date only four weeks away, I realize I could really do with a professional to talk to. But my old therapist is back in London, and it feels too late in the day to put something in place up here. I reassure myself that I don't feel as desperate as before. Being pregnant, however hard I am finding it, is clearly better than the alternative. Underneath the shrill notes of panic, there is a bass chord of happiness, of optimism, for every day I am still pregnant and can still feel the baby moving. It's just that it's easier to feel that deep, resonant thrum in some moments than in others. Like the blazing afternoon I decide to wash a first – modest – batch of newborn clothes. As I hang the half-dozen tiny white bodysuits out to dry, I can feel joy singing in my veins. By comparison, the nightmares drown it out, leaving me unsettled and full of nervous energy I have no satisfactory way of burning off, hindered by my increasingly improbable size and shape.

And then one day, I have a different kind of dream. I see Dan carrying our baby upstairs, bringing them to me to be fed. It is so detailed and true-to-life, from the grain of our wooden staircase to Dan's increasingly overgrown lockdown beard, that it feels more like a premonition. I see a small arm flailing against Dan's chest, as he ascends slowly; as slowly as if he were carrying a laden tea tray and doesn't want to spill a drop. I see a shock of dark hair and tightly curled fingers. There is no surprise ending to the scene. No heart-lurching twist. When I wake up, I feel as though I know what it is like to touch those fingers, to stroke that tiny head of hair. I try to hold on to the image for days afterwards. I let my mind relax around it just a little, leaning into the stretch. Maybe, just maybe, it really is going to work out this time.

13

'They'll come when they're ready'

(July 2020 – 40 weeks pregnant)

The morning after my due date, my waters break. At least, I think that's what it is. It happens as I heave one leg and then the other over the side of the bath to take a shower. At first, I wonder – with not a little humiliation – whether I have wet myself. But the liquid seems too clear for that. Then it happens again, as I stand washing my hair. Water is already cascading down my back, pouring off the preposterous dome of my stomach, but there is no mistaking this extra trickle and where it's come from.

I have been having niggling, stretching pains across my abdomen for a few days now. A couple of times, some unseen force pulled at me so tightly I was convinced that was it: labour. But the cramps never amounted to anything; no regular pattern emerged. I'd bounce on my Swiss ball as we watched telly, or I'd lumber into a different position in bed to try to get back to sleep, in expectation of the rigours to come – only they never did. Anticipation would evaporate, leaving behind stale impatience.

It is only in this last week that I have adjusted to actively want-ing pregnancy to end. When, for nearly ten months, your sole, clenched focus has been willing your body to stay pregnant, to start to wish for the opposite feels transgressive and disorient-ing. For so long I've lived with *not yet, not yet, not yet* that it is hard to fully compute that it's finally time: *now. Please, let it be now.*

Midwives and doulas sometimes refer to these final weeks and days of pregnancy as *zwischen*, a German word literally meaning 'between' but which in some contexts can convey a sense of impermanence, or of something being penultimate. *Inzwischen*, meaning 'meanwhile', can also be a way of suggesting a change between two different periods of time. In the words of Jana Studelska, the midwife who first co-opted the word to capture the peculiarity of this part of pregnancy, *zwischen* is 'the time and place where mothers linger, waiting to be called forward'. For anyone about to give birth, it's a phase that feels both tense and portentous. You cannot go back to who you were before and you cannot rush ahead to your future, either. In *zwischen*, you are standing at the unseen entrance to another world. Only you do not know when you will be allowed to cross. You also do not know *how* you will be enabled to cross. You are marooned in time, caught in the perpetual present, and yet it's knowing that things could change at any moment that gives that illusion. For me, adding to the surreal quality of these final days is how my desires now are an exact and unnerving counterpoint to the rest of my pregnancy. Whereas before I'd prayed that any slight twinge or ache would dissipate without incident, now I long for insistent cramps and contractions. Now, whenever I go to the bathroom, I am actively hoping to see some sign of wetness, or a trace of blood as the cervix softens – the very things I once dreaded. If *zwischen* is a hinterland, after miscarriage it can be one filled with ghosts and uncanny valleys.

After my shower, I put a sanitary pad in my underwear and

consult with Dan. We decide to give it half an hour and then we will call the hospital. I leak again. Triage tells me, once again, to come in. They will check whether it is amniotic fluid or 'something else'. The voice on the end of the phone spares me the indignity of them saying 'or just a wee'.

As we prepare ourselves to drive to the maternity unit, something else starts to gnaw at me. The baby seems quiet again. I know I have felt them moving this morning. But the kicks have been more spaced apart and seem to collide with my insides with less force than usual. Or am I imagining it? From the car, the world seems quiet, too. Even for a Sunday, it feels sleepier than normal. Dan has the radio tuned to a station called Mellow Magic, which plays a lot of unthreatening ballads and retro love songs. It has been, I think, his way of trying to keep us both as calm as possible on these types of journey. Usually, I would take my chance to tease him about his musical taste and the kind of thing he considers 'an absolute classic'. This time, though, the sentimental songs reduce me to tears. I don't feel sad, exactly. I am, on balance, less worried than on previous trips to the hospital. I'm crying because I am struck by the possibility that this could be the last time we'll do this. This could be the last time we drive to the hospital, with me still pregnant. More to the point, this could be a good thing.

Knowing when a baby is going to arrive is an imprecise science. Right from the beginning of your pregnancy, you are given an estimated due date, yet only 4 per cent of babies actually arrive on this assigned day. Research has suggested that just over half (55 per cent) of babies arrive within seven days either side of their estimated due date, and a not-insignificant 30 per cent arrive more than ten days either side of their due date. Due dates are typically calculated as being forty weeks or 280 days from the first day of your last period. This calculation is based on a more-than-200-year-old formula called Naegele's rule, after Franz Naegele, a German obstetrician who, in 1812, concluded you could reasonably predict when a woman would give birth by adding nine months and seven days on to the date her last period started. While Naegele's rule is what most online due-date calculators still work from, doctors and midwives today will also use ultrasound scans to date pregnancies and recalculate the due date if necessary, on the basis that someone may not remember their period dates perfectly, or they may have much shorter or longer cycles than the average twenty-eight days, and so could have ovulated and conceived earlier or later than the calculation presumes.

Even so, our reliance on Naegele's rule in the first place comes from a fundamental absence in our knowledge: we are unable to know for certain when conception takes place. As obstetrician Nick Macklon puts it to me, we only use the dates of someone's period as a proxy for when pregnancy began because, for most people who conceive naturally, we have no other way of knowing this. Even when doctors and researchers adapt Naegele's rule to try to calculate from ovulation, rather than a woman's last period, this is still not the precise moment pregnancy begins. Rather, it is presumed that conception, if it takes place, happens twenty-four hours later. 'One of the holy grails in this field, I think, would be if we had a marker of an embryo being in the uterus before it's even started implanting,' Professor Macklon tells me. At the moment, he adds, this is something we cannot observe or pinpoint, except in people undergoing IVF. Not only would this be useful for research into early pregnancy (and, therefore, miscarriage), it's possible that what happens in those very earliest moments of pregnancy has implications for its final moments. In 2013, a team of US researchers found that not only did the natural length of pregnancy seem to vary by as much as five weeks, but it seemed to vary according to what happened right at the start of pregnancy, such as how long it took for a fertilized egg to implant in the lining of the womb. In other words, 'the trajectory for

the timing of delivery may be set in early pregnancy', as reproductive epidemiologist Anne Marie Jukic, who led the study,
said at the time. Dr Jukic and her team had set out to investigate why there seems to be such a deviation in pregnancy length
and why due dates, according to the conventional formula, can
be so wide of the mark. This variation, the researchers noted in
the write-up of the study, is sometimes put down to errors in
estimating the age of a pregnancy according to period dates or
scans, so they wanted to test whether this was actually the case.

To do this, they used data from an existing study that closely
monitored women who were trying to conceive, analysing
their hormone levels in daily urine samples for six months or
until they became pregnant. This data pinpoints both ovulation and implantation, when the pregnancy hormone HCG
starts to be released (and days before it would be picked up by a
home pregnancy test). The researchers then used this information to give the precise length, in days, of any subsequent
pregnancies. Even when they excluded premature deliveries,
they found women's pregnancies varied in length by as much
as thirty-seven days. Because they'd measured the starts of
women's pregnancies so precisely, they concluded that this had
to be down to natural variation rather than any kind of error.
What's more, they noted that some women had a longer gap
between ovulation and implantation than others (it can take
anything from around six to twelve days) and these women
generally had longer pregnancies, as measured from the time of
implantation. On the other hand, women whose progesterone
production took longer to kick in were found to be more likely
to have a shorter-than-average pregnancy – twelve days shorter
than the median.[1] It is not the only time researchers have suggested that a 200-year-old formula might not be the best science
to go by in the twenty-first century. The idea that a single
rule to predict pregnancy length can apply to every pregnant
woman, regardless of her age, race, and pregnancy history,

'stretches credulity', according to consultant obstetrician Gerald Wightman Lawson, who published an analysis of available data on due dates and pregnancy length in 2021.[2]

It may seem like common sense that pregnancies would naturally vary in length. After all, as a species we vary widely in almost everything from height and build to pain tolerance. And despite being assigned a nominal due date, most women understand that in reality there's a broad range of possible birthdays for their baby. However, a desire to know any more than this, to try to divine whether you, personally, will deliver early, late, or right on schedule, is often met with short shrift. Pregnancy books and blogs repeatedly remind you that the onset of labour is an unknown quantity. Any expectation to the contrary is, it is insinuated, naive or even prima donna-ish. 'They'll come when they are good and ready' is a common sentiment. 'You're on your baby's schedule now – welcome to parenting!' is another. Case closed, discussion over. Who do we think we are to expect such precise, rational information about our bodies?

Yet this barely concealed paternalism skips blithely over gaps in our knowledge. Not least, the rather elemental question: why does labour begin in the first place? The short answer is 'we just don't know', Professor Andrew Shennan, an obstetrician and director of the Tommy's Preterm Birth Surveillance Clinic at Guy's and St Thomas' Hospital in London, tells me. There are well-known signs that labour could be imminent – but we do not know exactly what kicks the whole thing off. Signs that labour might not be far away include: the baby moving into a favourable position, with the head moving further down inside the pelvis; a bloody 'show' as the cervix starts to soften, the jelly-like plug of mucus that protects the womb from infection possibly coming away and passing out of the vagina; waters breaking; and the onset of mild contractions and/or backache. Yet there is a huge variability in how women experience these things. Sometimes they happen weeks before someone gives birth; sometimes it is mere moments before active labour begins. They do not necessarily happen in a particular order. They do not necessarily happen at all. It's yet another example of how 'we don't know' is taken as a sufficient answer when it comes to women's bodies.

There are a few clues, from population data and studies, to whether you are more likely to deliver early or go overdue. Weight may have an influence. 'There's some evidence that women who are obese will labour later, because there are biological reasons why obesity might prevent or delay spontaneous onset of labour,' explains Professor Shennan. 'There's a substance called leptin, which is produced by fat cells, for example, which has effects on the uterus's ability to contract.' It's also thought that those who conceive through IVF are more likely to go beyond their due date, although it is not clear why this should be. Based on current available evidence, one of the strongest predictors of when you, personally, will go into labour seems to be your family history. For example, if you have a sister who went overdue, you are more likely to do so as well. Likewise, if you went overdue last time, it's more likely you will again. A baby's biological father and his family history may make a difference, too.[3]

Recognizing that 'current methods to predict spontaneous labour are fairly inaccurate', a team of researchers at the Prematurity Research Center at Stanford University, California, are working on a simple blood test that could help pinpoint when someone is likely to give birth. In 2021, they published the results of a study that found there was a particular signature of physical changes in a woman's blood around three weeks before labour starts. They analysed blood samples of pregnant women for 7,142 different biomarkers, including immune cells and hormones, and found that as women moved into this pre-labour phase, their blood showed a distinct increase in progesterone and cortisol, as well as a drop in factors that help blood vessel formation, and a rise in substances that are needed for blood-clotting (possibly to help prevent blood loss during and after delivery).[4] There were also notable changes to the activity of immune-system proteins, in particular one called IL-1R4, which inhibits inflammation. Scientists have theorized for a while that labour is triggered by some sort of immune response. However, based on these new findings, as one of the Stanford researchers, Virginia Winn, explained, 'it's not a single switch; there's this preparation that the body has to go through'. Critically, this shift was independent of gestational age and the same pattern was detected both in women who gave birth at full term and women who delivered prematurely. The Stanford team's hope is that they will now be able to refine their work in order to come up with a straightforward test that doctors can easily use during pregnancy. Potentially, they've said, this could happen within the next two to three years, which could be reassuring for many.

There are important reasons for wanting to know more about when and why labour starts – reasons that have little to do with a desire to micromanage all of the mystery and magic in our lives. Being able to establish whether someone is imminently at risk of going into premature labour could allow doctors to take steps to give a baby the best chance of survival, such as administering steroids to help mature their lungs, for example. Being able to know how far off labour actually is could also help to answer a question that dominates the final days of pregnancy for an increasing number of women: whether to have labour artificially induced.

At the hospital, this is the choice that awaits me.

'As you're now forty weeks, we can induce you – if you want?' The doctor's voice is crisp, but kind. She's looking at me intently, through her fashionable, thick-rimmed glasses, as though she's trying to read my mind.

'We could even start it tonight,' she says again, before adding

quickly, 'if that's what you want?' It's been determined that my
waters have not, in fact, broken. A swab of the contents of my
sanitary pad suggests it is not amniotic fluid. The baby's heart
rate is also found to be OK. However, as this is my third time
at the unit with worries about reduced movements, a consultant has been summoned to review my notes and to talk to me
about my options.

I look down at my shoes. I'm unsure how to explain to her
what I'm thinking.

'You don't have to have the induction,' the consultant continues. 'You could go home, but in that case we'd suggest you
come back tomorrow for another scan, just to keep an eye on
things.'

Oh.

I'm not sure if I want the induction, but, I realize, I don't
really want to go home either. When she'd uttered the word
induction, my immediate reaction – a feeling, more than a
thought – had been relief. Warm, cosseting relief, like sinking
into a bath. I wouldn't have to wait any more. At least with an
induction, I think, there will be a change of scene, and something else to think about. But a wave of doubt rolls in fast
behind. Induced labour is supposed to be a thing you resist,
that you don't want – isn't it?

I have not seen fit to make a birth plan. I have not explicitly
ruled out induction. I have no particular attachment to a 'natural'
birth, whatever that even really means.* And a conviction has
been building since this morning that this pregnancy has run its
course – though whether that comes from some instinct about
the well-being of my pregnancy or whether it is anxiety finally

---

* 'Natural' and 'normal' are generally used as stand-ins for 'vaginal' birth – a more
specific word that newspapers and healthcare professionals alike are often still
strangely reluctant to use – as opposed to a caesarean section, though, of course,
for some purists you can only lay claim to a 'natural' birth if you decline all interventions and pain relief.

getting the better of me, I am less sure. What's more, there is a small, sneaky voice wheedling that an induction is a coward's way out. That it is not 'real' childbirth. I'm surprised and disappointed that I think this. After four years and four miscarriages, I thought I had escaped the pressure of aspiring to a particular kind of birth. For me, birth was just a means to an end. But apparently not. Could this unfamiliar voice be right? If I say yes, if I allow myself to be led up to the antenatal ward right now, will I be denying myself some fullness of this experience? More seriously, could I be setting myself up for failure and unnecessary trauma?

There are very valid reasons for wanting to avoid an induced labour, which typically involves having the cervix softened or 'ripened' using a pessary or gel containing hormone-like substances called prostaglandins, followed by the amniotic sac being broken manually, then a drip of a synthetic form of the hormone oxytocin to stimulate contractions. They are widely acknowledged to lead to a more painful labour, possibly because the synthetic form of oxytocin used doesn't cross into the brain in the same way that the natural oxytocin a woman produces during spontaneous labour does, where it is believed to offer a degree of protection against pain and distress (oxytocin is sometimes referred to as the 'cuddle' or 'love' hormone, because of its role in sex, physical touch, and social bonding). However, this is all hypothetical, rather than something that's been tested and proven. Inductions have also been linked with greater use of other interventions during labour, such as forceps, ventouse (a suction device), or having an episiotomy (cutting the tissue between the vaginal opening and the anus to create more space) to aid delivery, each of which in turn is associated with vaginal tearing and damage to the pelvic floor muscles. Women are also often told that induced labours are more likely to end in an unplanned caesarean than spontaneous labours are. In fact, a recent high-quality evidence review by the Cochrane group, which collated the data from thirty-four different studies, suggests that having an induction does not increase the risk of needing a caesarean, having an assisted delivery, or perineal trauma.[5] But it's undeniably true that opting for an induced labour often means giving birth in a particular kind of environment – usually in a hospital delivery suite. It may mean constant monitoring via a CTG machine* and frequent internal examinations, which many women would rather avoid.

Inductions are very common. One in three labours in the UK today are the result of an induction. Ten years ago, it was one in five. However, despite their increasingly widespread use, inductions are not a sure thing. Sometimes, they simply do not work, and it's not really known why. It's also difficult to gauge how likely it is that an induction will fail, with one recent study suggesting that just 2 per cent don't progress to active labour, while other sources suggest that this is the case for as many as 25 per cent of first-time mothers (who then, ultimately, need a caesarean). This is something that the kind of work being done at the Stanford Prematurity Center could help to shed light on. As the researchers working on blood biomarkers to predict labour pointed out, the baby being ready to be born is just one factor – the mother's body has to be ready, too. Yet this is the side of the equation that remains a relative mystery.

'There are a lot of women who, when you ask, will tell you that their experience of induction is very traumatic,' Professor Soo Downe, a midwife and an academic at the University of Central Lancashire, tells me. 'The difficulty is knowing whether that would also have been the case if they'd had a spontaneous labour.' Professor Downe is one of several authors of a recent study, published in 2021, that attempted to address this particular difficulty. Obviously, the same woman cannot give birth

---

* A cardiotocograph, which keeps track of a foetal heartbeat.

twice in the same pregnancy in order to provide a perfectly controlled comparison. However, you may be able to get a better idea of the differences between induction and spontaneous labour by comparing similar women, having similar pregnancies. For their study, therefore, Professor Downe, along with researchers from Western Sydney University and Amsterdam University Medical Centers, looked at data from almost 70,000 births where labour was induced for no specific medical reason. They found that for first-time mothers with uncomplicated pregnancies, being induced was much more likely to result in needing an epidural for the pain, an episiotomy, an unplanned caesarean section, or severe bleeding post-delivery (although the risk of that last one was still small – 2.4 per cent for induced labour versus 1.5 per cent for spontaneous labour).[6]

However, just what this means for women's long-term well-being, both physical and psychological, remains unknown. 'We've not really got the evidence yet,' says Professor Downe. Trying to unpick the psychological consequences of induced labour is 'complicated', she says. As it stands, there is no long-term data on how women actually feel after having had an induction as opposed to waiting for labour to start – or how it impacted their quality of life beyond the delivery room. It is a breathtaking absence. Once again, the hidden costs of what we don't know or haven't bothered to find out are potentially huge – and pregnant or recently pregnant women are expected to pick up the tab without complaint.

Of course, there is one very compelling reason doctors regularly offer and perform inductions – the reason they prefer not to let women go too far beyond their due date, and why an induction can be offered at the first hint of trouble, be it reduced movements, signs of a baby's growth slowing down, or gestational diabetes. Inducing labour early is one of the few strategies doctors have for preventing stillbirth. In November 2021, NICE (the National Institute for Health and Care Excellence) updated its guidance to recommend that all women in England should be offered an induction by forty-one weeks of pregnancy – a week overdue. This was a full week earlier than the previous advice. The change followed several large studies that showed a small but significant increase in the risk of still-birth as pregnancy goes on, after someone has reached full term (thirty-seven weeks). In 2019, a British study that analysed data from 15 million pregnancies calculated that the risk of stillbirth rose incrementally from 0.11 in 1,000 pregnancies at thirty-seven weeks to more than three in 1,000 by forty-two weeks. Then there was a Swedish trial, the results of which were pub-lished the same year, that had to be halted early on ethical grounds after six babies died in the group of women selected to be induced at forty-two weeks as opposed to forty-one weeks. 'In my opinion, this was sadly entirely predictable, based on what we already knew,' obstetrician Professor Alexander Heazell tells me.

Professor Heazell is director of the Rainbow Clinic at St Mary's Hospital in Manchester, a specialist unit researching stillbirth and neonatal death. The clinic is part-funded by the charity Tommy's and sees people from all over the UK who have lost babies late on in pregnancy, or during or shortly after birth. Some patients have endured this wrenching, primal kind of loss multiple times. Clinically speaking, stillbirth – like recurrent miscarriage – is considered rare. In high-income countries, it affects around one in 200 pregnancies. In the UK, seven babies a day are stillborn and, in 2020, 2,638 families lost their baby this way. Of course, whether that sounds like a remote possibility to you is all a matter of perspective and pre-vious experience. Yet in mainstream pregnancy advice there can be a deep reluctance to engage with the subject. The word 'stillbirth' is often avoided altogether, its possibility sema-phored instead through phrases like 'at risk', 'not looking right', or 'baby's a bit unhappy'. Measures to prevent stillbirth – such as new, evidence-based advice to go to sleep on your side during the final trimester[7] – are still airily dismissed by some midwives as scaremongering.

For many babies who are stillborn, there is no obvious or identifiable cause – even after a hospital post-mortem examination. There is likely no single cause of stillbirth; however, there is a hypothesis that one factor could be the placenta becoming less efficient as pregnancy waxes on. Some researchers have suggested that the placenta ages – possibly at different rates between different women – and that at a certain point a mismatch develops between the needs of the growing baby and the ability of the placenta to transfer oxygen and nutrients, with potentially fatal consequences. This is why there is so much interest and debate around when to induce women as they approach the end of their pregnancy.

Yet, says Professor Heazell, this is not always something women are made aware of. 'I do see women who've had stillbirths after forty or forty-one weeks – even as late as forty-three weeks – and they always say nobody told them this could happen; nobody had a proper conversation with them,' he tells me. 'Nobody tells them the risk is higher after forty-one weeks than at forty weeks.' Sometimes, he adds, women are told they need an induction, but the specific nature of the risk is kept vague, the word stillbirth unsaid. 'If we can't articulate why, it's no wonder that women will decline the offer,' Professor Heazell reflects. Equally, the reluctance to utter the word 'stillbirth' and spell out the rationale behind inductions – to explain the actual level of risk potentially involved – can actually cause more panic. 'It can come across as a doctor or midwife saying: "If you don't do as I say, your baby will die,"' Professor Heazell adds. In my own online antenatal classes, I noted the conspicuous absence of the word 'stillbirth' as the tutor started to talk us through the potential risks and complications of having an induced labour. Having written a piece on inductions for a newspaper a few months previously, I waited for her to explain the logic behind offering them in the first place. I listened carefully. The word never once came out of her mouth.

When it comes to induction, Professor Heazell says: 'There isn't a right or wrong answer, because it comes down to what individual women feel are the right things to do. There are some women who will say, "That's a remote possibility. I don't want an induction." In which case, that's fine, that's an educated decision. What isn't fine, in my view, is a professional deciding that a one in 200 risk is remote, so they're not even going to discuss it with someone.'

Inducing lots of people, who may not want or need such an intervention, to reduce the overall number of stillborn babies is an undeniably blunt tool. It's been estimated that 426 extra inductions have to be performed in order to prevent one perinatal death (this includes stillborn babies, as well as maternal deaths, or babies who die shortly after birth). The fundamental dilemma here comes down to the same thing: what we still don't know about the pregnant body. There isn't yet an easy or reliable way to tell whose baby is actually at risk from an ageing placenta and who is likely to be fine to go beyond their due date. Many different strategies to prevent stillbirth, such as offering additional scans in the third trimester or improving awareness of foetal movements among pregnant women and/or hospital staff, have, unfortunately, been found to make no meaningful difference in trials so far.[8] It may be that in the near future we will be able to tell whether the placenta is deteriorating from a blood test. Australian research, for example, has identified particular molecular and cellular changes in placental tissue that suggest 'senescence' – that is, ageing tissue.[9] Meanwhile, in the UK there are ongoing attempts to identify biomarkers in blood that point to placental dysfunction.[10] Until we unlock more of the biology, though, women will have to rely on probability and judgement alone.

As for what's right for me, right now, I have no idea. I'm

sitting back in the car with Dan, clutching a sheaf of information from the consultant. As relieved as I am at the thought they could induce me today, I'm also aware that my perception of risk is, by dint of experience, wildly out of kilter. How worried – and therefore proactive – should I be? What does today's drop-off in movements really mean? What about the earlier concerns about the baby's growth? On a strictly rational prospectus, do I qualify as someone for whom there is no medical need to induce? Or have there been potential signs that my pregnancy is, to a greater or lesser extent, on borrowed time? Even if it could be proven beyond all doubt that there is no pressing physical need, does my state of mind count for nothing, here?

I have no blueprint for reaching this decision. A history of miscarriage is treated as largely irrelevant when it comes to giving birth. And yet it transforms the entire inner landscape of pregnancy and how you make every, infinitesimal decision. It is also not physically irrelevant, either. Recurrent miscarriage is a 'sentinel risk marker' for obstetric complications, such as pre-term birth, but also for placental abruption and foetal growth restriction, according to the authors of a paper published in the *Lancet* in 2021. The same research paper, which reviewed all the existing literature, suggested that the risk of perinatal complications rises with the number of previous pregnancy losses, too.[11] Although I do not know this yet. No one, at any point in my pregnancy so far, has mentioned anything like it.

I can feel the pull of what I am supposed to want in this situation. There is part of me that wants to linger in the fantasy life of being a person whose biggest concern about labour is whether or not they will get to use the birthing pool. Wrapped around this small fragment of make-believe is a notion that by doing things a certain way – by trying to think the way I would have thought before my miscarriages – perhaps I can make up for lost time. Perhaps I can get back to that version of myself

who knew exactly what brand of pram she wanted and the specific shade she was going to paint the nursery. She would, I
think, have had very fixed ideas about the kind of birth that
was 'best'. She would have felt confident in her choices; invin-
cible. There would, I suspect, have been a plan. It would have
involved yogic breathing and candles. Not bright hospital lights
and constant monitoring: someone and something else keeping
a close eye on that heartbeat – the heartbeat we've waited so
long to hear. There's that warm-bath feeling again.

It is fashionable to talk about having a 'positive' birth. It's
supposed to mean that someone makes their own choices about
location, who is with them, pain relief and any other medical
interventions, based on accurate information, leaving them
feeling in control, powerful, and respected. It shouldn't be controversial to say that a positive birth could just as easily mean a
candle-lit homebirth as a planned caesarean, depending on the
person, depending on the circumstances. And yet, all too often,
only certain kinds of choices are seen as 'positive' ones, while
others are painted as mere capitulation. What counts as a positive birth, for someone like me? Is such a thing even possible?
In this moment, I just don't know. A tenet of 'positive' birth is
that decisions should be made based on reality, rather than from
fear. But fear *is* my reality.

There is hardly any published research on the feelings and
attitudes of women giving birth after miscarriage. I can find
nothing at all on labour after recurrent miscarriage. It's a perspective that's hard to locate in mainstream writing about
birth, too. In the last two weeks of my pregnancy, having
reached the uncomfortable bargain with my anxiety that,
whatever happened, I was still going to have to give birth, I
read it all. I read the practical-advice books by modern, prac-
tising NHS midwives. I read the uncannily similar and serene
birth stories of lifestyle bloggers. I read cult classics on natural

childbirth by Second Wave activist-midwifes, with their emphasis on the mind/body connection and tales of orgasmic birth. And I read the data-driven defences of having an epidural. I find a line in Ina May Gaskin's *Guide to Childbirth* that suggests 'a woman who has had a miscarriage . . . already has some life training that should help her give birth without becoming terribly frightened of pain itself'. But that's about it. Once again, I feel stateless; caught between two sides of a debate. The renowned midwife and natural-childbirth advocate Sheila Kitzinger wrote that the labouring woman must 'have learned to trust her body and its instincts'. But this is anathema to someone like me, who feels that their body has let them down again and again. No matter how many reassuring hypnobirthing tracks I listen to, how physically fit and strong I feel, or how unafraid of the pain, the mistrust in my body's ability to give me a baby is something I cannot reframe. Equally, I can take only a partial comfort in Western medicine's power to intervene. Miscarriage, after all, shows you both its limitations and its indifference.

I decide to call my mum. Mum, I know, has had both induced and non-induced labours. True to form, she doesn't mince her words.

'I'd just go for it, if I were you.'

An induction might take a while to get going, she warns me. It might also mean the actual labour is pretty intense, but she reckons I can handle it. She tells me all this in the sort of considered, factful tone she might use to talk me through a complicated recipe. Then she pauses, and something shifts.

'I think you're too anxious to go home now.'

I can picture the exact expression on her face as she says this. It's a penetrating look I recognize as her working out something about me that I've not quite worked out for myself. This makes me cry again. She's right. I am too anxious to go home.

I cannot wait any more. And that's OK. I feel my head bobbing in agreement.

'I'm nodding,' I say, remembering she can't see me.

'It's time,' Mum says.

'You've got the whole place to yourself,' a midwife tells me brightly as she leads me upstairs to the antenatal ward, where she's going to give me the first pessary to get the induction started. Dan has gone home to fetch my things. Just *my* bag; not the bag I've packed for the baby. Not yet. Dan will be allowed to stay for a little while this evening, to keep me company, but not overnight.

I have never known a hospital ward as still and silent as this one. There is no bustle, no bleeping of machines or rattle of passing trolleys. There are no other footsteps in the corridor. It's a ghost town, I think. And then I wish that particular phrase had not sprung to mind.

'You should have seen it two weeks ago,' the midwife tells me as she opens the door to my room. 'We'd never been so busy – I've only just recovered!' She widens her eyes for comic effect.

I feel a rush of gratitude for the enveloping quiet, realizing that it might not always have been this way. This is something else we rarely talk about when it comes to birth: the many factors beyond our control, dictated by politics, geography, funding, and sheer luck of the draw; the healthcare system your particular country operates under; how busy the hospital is that particular day. As the essayist Leslie Jamison puts it, there is an uncomfortable truth at the heart of anyone's labour experience: 'it feels deeply personal but has in fact been shaped by impersonal societal forces'. During and after pregnancy, our conversations circle endlessly around what we choose and do for ourselves, crediting our decisions for what goes right and blaming ourselves for what goes wrong. We may not wish to dwell on the ways we are at the mercy of the system or how maternity care is organized where we live, but that doesn't change the fact that we are. We rarely consider the things that might have the biggest impact of all – things we could actually change as a society. Like the fact that England is short of almost 2,500 midwives. Or how, according to one recent survey, eight out of ten midwives feel there are typically not enough staff on shift to provide a safe service. The Royal College of Midwives' chief executive Gill Walton also said in 2021 that 'not a day goes by' without a report of a maternity unit somewhere in the country being closed temporarily and patients diverted elsewhere due to lack of staff. 'Continuity of care' – that is, seeing a midwife who knows you and your history throughout pregnancy – has been shown to reduce the risk of stillbirth, as well as premature birth, according to a 2016 Cochrane review of data from 17,674 pregnancies.[12] Staff shortages also have an unseen impact on pregnancy research, when studies require women to be enrolled from labour wards or other clinical settings. Because when midwives and doctors are pushed to the brink, talking people through study protocols, gaining consent, and completing extra paperwork is, inevitably – understandably – going to take a backseat. Would I be here, in my own room, feeling unrushed and well attended, had this happened a fortnight ago? Would I even have been offered this induction at all?

Despite getting to the hospital around midday, the afternoon has slipped away from us. It's well past dinner time and I'm brought a cheese sandwich and a strawberry yoghurt, thin and synthetically sweet, but not unpleasant. By the time Dan returns with my bags, there is not long before he has to leave again. I'm told to try to sleep for a few hours before someone will be in to examine my cervix and 'pop' me on the monitor. It'll be the middle of the night, but I find I don't mind. It feels both exciting and comforting. I feel more at peace than I have

in weeks. So, this is where my *zwischen* will end. This is what
the portal to that other realm will look like for me: a small,
square room with a slanting ceiling, somewhere on the first
floor of a city hospital. From my bathroom window, I can see
the maze of corridors and annexes that make up the maternity
unit and triage below, and a slice of lilac sky above. The stars
are not yet out. Just before I drift off to sleep, I hear the start of
rain pittering against the roof. It has been threatening to break
all day.

I'd been told it could take as long as three days for the induced
contractions to start – and for the really hard work to begin.
But things get going quickly. Too quickly.

Even before Dan has arrived back at the hospital in the morning, I'm told that my uterus is responding 'a little too well'.
There is a concern it could be hyperstimulated, as the monitor
suggests my contractions, which started around dawn, are coming very close together. I'd been warned there was a risk of this
last night. Apart from being intensely painful, hyperstimulation can also affect the baby's heart rate, cause foetal distress,
and in extreme cases risks rupturing the uterine muscles. It can
mean an induction has to be halted. Sometimes the baby will
have to be delivered by emergency caesarean section. However,
I had been reassured that it hardly ever happens.

'I can't remember the last time I saw a case,' the cheery midwife had said.

I'm both surprised and not surprised. I never assume something 'rare' won't happen to me any more. Also, something is
starting to crystallize for me: perhaps this is just what my body
does. It goes in too hard, too fast, too eager. Ever the try-hard.
It conceives when it shouldn't. It responds too well to the medication. What is surprising, however, is that I feel essentially fine.
Reassuringly, the baby's heart rate also seems untroubled. A lot
of the contractions the monitor is apparently picking up barely

register on my own internal scale. Stones skimming across a lake. Even the contractions I do feel – the rocks that do break the surface – are certainly no more painful than my first two miscarriages. And the flesh-memory of those particular contractions makes this seem easier. As much as the pain grips and bites, my muscles seeming to be pushed in one direction while pulled in another, at least this feels constructive in a way that miscarriage pains cannot. Remembering the abject hopelessness of those cramps, the pointlessness of that blood, calms me. Whatever this is, it is not yet like that. *We are still in the game.*

At 2 p.m., I am taken down to the delivery suite, as I am deemed to be dilated enough to have my waters broken manually. I don't really feel the actual piercing, but there is no doubt that it has happened. Liquid pours out of me. And it strikes me as quite funny that I mistook what happened yesterday morning in the shower for my waters breaking: there is just so much of it. For a while, things remain calm. All my thoughts, hopes, and worries seem to retreat. They are gathered together, somewhere deep inside me. I watch TV on my iPad and flick through a book. Dan goes to the hospital canteen for snacks. He sends some work emails. Then the midwives decide it is time to move on to the final stage of the induction – the hormone drip.

Soon after, I stop being able to read or watch the sitcom episodes I'd downloaded. There is no room for narrative now, only sensation. Staying still is also not an option. Time starts playing tricks. The wrench of my contractions seems to go on for ever, only stopping just when I think I can take no more. Then the minutes in between flit by at double speed. I breathe, trying to keep in time with an app on my phone. I change position. I breathe. I change position. Time stops. I change position. Time stops again. At the last check, I was only 2cm dilated. This means I have hours to go yet. But I am increasingly agitated. Dan rubs my shoulders. I'm struggling to keep hold of my breath, to hold the numbers in my head to count with. He counts for me. He presses his hands down gently on my shoulders. I sit on my Swiss ball, with my back against his knees. I stand with my hands on my hips. I circle them. I rock. I lean forward. I lean against the wall. Then time starts to shudder and skip.

I'm back on the bed. I'm not sure how that happened. Would I like to try the gas and air, now? Actually, no, I would like to die, thank you very much. Dan holds the nozzle of the gas and air, because I find I cannot grip it for myself. It expands inside me. I feel dizzy. But it is not enough. I suck and gulp again. And I'm not even halfway, I think, in a fleeting lucid moment.

'Jennifer,' I hear the midwife say, calling to me from the opposite end of a long tunnel. 'Do you feel like you want to push, Jennifer?'

That's exactly what I want, I think, relieved. And then I'm over on my hands and knees. I push and I push. Over and over. Again and again. It could be minutes. It could be days. Someone tells me I am nearly there. Someone else tells me they can see the head. Now they can feel the hair. Then they make me stop pushing, briefly. They tell me they need to attach a clip to the baby's head to be able to keep track of the heart rate. They try, but they cannot get the electrode to stick to the emerging scalp. They try again, but it's still not working. And I cannot hold on any longer; I will burst at the seams. Momentarily, it occurs to me that we are flying blind now, the baby and me. There is no way of knowing what is happening to its heart rate. I experience this thought with gleaming clarity, but without panic. There is no longer any space in my body for fear. I push and I push again. Again and again and again, until something releases. There is more liquid, and falling. Slipperiness. And then there he is, on the bed underneath me. A *he*.

Air becomes breath.

'The baby' becomes our son.

My first impression of our boy is that he is reddish-grey and absolutely livid with us. His reedy, panicked screams fill the room. To me, it feels as though he cries instantly – as if he knows that what I have been most afraid of is silence at this point and so he chooses to come out bawling. But Dan will tell me later that it was the single longest moment of his life, waiting for noise from those new, new lungs. It is the most beautiful sound I have ever heard. As he yells and yells, the many ghostly visions I've had of how this moment might play out disperse. There is no crash cart. No sudden descent of people into the room. My boy is not whisked away, limp and silent. Relief is pulsing through me. I am both more exhausted and more energized than I have ever been. I want to laugh and dance and cry and sleep.

'It's OK,' I murmur to my boy as the midwife places him on my chest. 'It's OK. It's OK.' I repeat it over and over and over, a reflex from a place beyond thought. I say it like saying grace. I say it like a catechism. I say it because, for the first time in a long time, I actually believe it.

14

'Enjoy every minute'

(July 2020 – 6 hours old)

Motherhood is incredible. It is 2 a.m. and I am supposed to be sleeping, but instead I'm sitting up on my bed in the postnatal ward, just watching my son's chest rise and fall. He is sleeping. I am euphoric. He's lying in a clear plastic cot, which I've already moved as close to me as possible. The extra 30cm the midwife had left between our beds felt much, much too far. His eyes and fists are tightly scrunched against this new, enormous world. There is a sheen of white wax across his nose and the skin along his eyebrows is flaking slightly. There is also the merest glaze of blood – whether his or mine, I do not know. Inside a complicated origami arrangement of towels and blankets, he wears a striped sleepsuit: thin grey lines stencilled across pristine white, like the rules of a brand-new exercise book. He looks nothing like I'd pictured. His hair is fine, and almost sandy – not thick and dark like mine. He is a revelation and also wholly familiar. I know him by heart.

Who could sleep at a time like this? Who could bear to miss a single moment?

Motherhood is terrifying. I need to rewrap the blankets around the baby, but I'm unsure how. I can't remember the exact configuration they were in before – and it seems significant. What if there's a dangerous way to wrap blankets? What if I don't do it right and he suffocates? The midwife parcelled him up in the delivery suite, but I didn't see how she did it. Dan was the one to dress the baby, as I was still having my reluctant placenta tugged out of me by a doctor. I watched, my head on the bed, as the midwife coached my husband through putting the first nappy, then the vest and babygrow, on our son. Dan's movements had been slow and self-conscious, as if the baby were a thing that might break.

Had the midwife shown *him* the right way to wrap the blankets? Why don't I know? Isn't this the kind of thing mothers are meant to know?

Around 4 a.m., I had to change the baby's nappy. What looked like black tar was everywhere: on the cot sheet; down his legs. It was hard to see what I was doing, and I was afraid to turn on too many lights in case I woke the woman in the bed opposite. An unfamiliar midwife on the nightshift bustled in to help, deploying wipes and getting a new nappy on with such speed and competence that I'd stepped back and just watched, limply. Only, she didn't re-do the blanket burrito before she left and now I don't know what to do. I'm starting to panic. I really don't want to get this wrong. I stick my head beyond the wipe-clean cubicle curtain, craning to see into the main corridor, in case the midwife is still there. The ward receptionist sees me.

'Do you want the midwife?'

I nod meekly.

'What for?'

I blink at her. Then I try to explain. Only the words come out garbled and back to front. I am swaying slightly on the spot, just barely aware of my own addled state. So, I *am* tired, after all. Her face hardens, an amalgam of scorn and annoyance.

'It's your baby. You can do it however you want.'

I go back to my bed. Daylight is just starting to creep through the cubicle curtain, leaving a blueish cast across my son's skin. He looks deathly; asphyxiated. I rest my hand lightly on his stomach to prove to myself he is still breathing. Then I tuck one end of the blanket under his armpits and wrap the other all the way around him. I don't want the covers to be too tight, but I am equally afraid of leaving them too loose. I am careful to keep them well away from his face and check there are no stray corners that might somehow migrate over his mouth and nose. But I still don't dare shut my eyes. I need to stay awake and watch him breathing, just in case. I'll wait for Dan to get here. He can take over the watch, then I will sleep.

Motherhood is blissful. After a day in hospital, we name our son Edward. Another night after that, we are allowed to come home. Cards and packages come to our door in a steady supply. Flowers spill out of every vase we own, even – at one point – a measuring jug. I catch myself gazing around the house in wonder. Every room feels bright and warm. I hang my son's implausibly tiny new dressing gown on the back of his bedroom door. I wash and put away his new clothes and arrange his new cuddly toys. His name starts to appear everywhere: stitched into blankets, stamped on to cards, inscribed on the flyleaves of books. I spend most mornings in bed, either feeding, or sleeping while Edward sleeps in his Moses basket beside me. The sheets on our bed are as white and vast as ships' sails. Without ever leaving the room, we are taking a wild voyage, this little stowaway and me. He is learning how to live in the world, how to feed, how some parts of the day are dark and others light.

Meanwhile, I am learning how to look after him outside of my body, yet still with my body. I am learning his rhythms and how to live on Edward-time, untethered. Sunlight bleeds through our bedroom curtains. Everything smells sweetly milky. Dan goes to register the birth. On various pieces of medical paperwork, I sign my name next to the box that says 'mother'. I have never felt so happy, so necessary, or so loved.

Motherhood is unbearable. Every time Edward cries, it is as if something detonates in my brain. A car alarm going off; a thousand sirens. In the evenings, especially, nothing seems to soothe him. He feeds and cries, feeds and cries. He cries if we put him down. He cries if we hold him. And I can't stand it. Not being able to give him what he needs is a physical sensation – my skin fizzes with it, my bones ache with it – and all the while the inside of my head screams. I am more tired than I have ever been and yet I cannot rest. Even when the house is silent, I hear Edward crying. Phantom cries interrupt just as I fumble for the edge of sleep. They convince me to step out of the shower, seconds after I've stepped in. On our fourth night home, while Dan rocks Edward yet again, pacing the length of our living room, I stand outside our front door in my pyjamas, staring up the lane, wanting to run into the cool, dark quiet. Instead, I fill my lungs with air, wrestle my panic back into its cage, and go back inside. Dan, I can't help feeling, copes so much better than I do in these moments. Although I know he is tired and frustrated too, he seems to stay so much calmer; he is so much more patient than me. I feel like I'm failing. I feel unnatural.

When Edward is ten days old, I spot a sore patch of skin under his armpit. It is oozing slightly, clearly infected. I show it to the midwife who comes to see us that morning. She agrees it looks like an infection, reassures us not to worry, but says we should call the out-of-hours GP to see if they can prescribe something. A video-call followed by an in-person appointment

later, and it is determined that, because of his age, Edward
needs to be admitted to the children's ward for intravenous
antibiotics right away. Pandemic restrictions mean only one
parent can stay with him. Because I am breastfeeding Edward –
or trying to – it has to be me. Dan is not allowed to visit, or
even come to the room to drop us off. By the time we get to the
hospital, something in my lower back is yelling, yanked out of
place from carrying Edward in his car seat.

They've said we will need to be in for at least forty-eight
hours. I am devastated, unsure how I will manage without Dan.
I watch, dazed, as the doctors hold my boy down on the bed
and insert a cannula into his tiny arm. Something inside me
collapses, seeing how vulnerable he looks, lying against the
pale-green hospital sheet, the eyes of an old man and the body
of a baby bird. The bandage they wrap around his arm afterwards is so large it will not fit in his sleepsuit. I have to leave him
half-dressed. His exposed upper arm is like a reproach. *Look:
how you have failed him.* Underneath this is a deeper terror. You
are constantly reminded, as a new parent, of the importance of
your own instincts – the fabled maternal instinct. But today, my
instincts got this completely wrong. I might have spotted the
infection, but as there was no other change in Edward, I assumed
it would be fine if I cleaned it up and put some nappy cream
over it. What if I hadn't mentioned it to the midwife? What if
the midwife hadn't happened to be visiting today? What if I'd
waited even twenty-four hours longer to see a doctor? I am
crushed by my own mistaken judgement. *I am terrible at this*, I
think. And then a layer beneath that: *This is because you were not
meant to be a mother.* The nurse who comes to check on Edward
in the middle of the night sees that I'm crying. I'm not sure
when I started – I think I may have been crying since we
arrived – but I cannot seem to stop. She speaks to me kindly,
trying to calm me down, but at the end of every clause she
doesn't use my name, she calls me 'mum': *'What's upset you,*

mum?' . . . *'Don't cry, mum'* . . . *'The thing is, mum'* . . . *'I know you're tired, mum'*. I know she's only trying to help, but I wish she'd stop. Every time she says it, I feel like I am disappearing.

Motherhood is everything I hoped it would be. Motherhood is also frightening, lonely, demoralizing. I feel complete. I feel torn apart. It is good and then it is bad again and then good again. It is complicated by my having wanted it so much. It is complicated by what has gone before. And yet motherhood is where the stories we tell about miscarriage tend to both start and stop. Often, people only speak about their early pregnancy losses once they have carried a baby to term and got on with the day-to-day business of being a mother; a family. The miscarriage stories we usually hear in the media are almost always told in hindsight, from this safe place of 'success'. What's more, that someone has gone on to have a healthy baby is often the last word on the matter – the pay-off line of an article, implying resolution and redemption. But a miscarriage, or miscarriages, are not necessarily felt as merely a 'blip' in a bigger journey; there can be lasting effects. Nor is motherhood a total cure for the experience. The paradox here is that while it may feel easier – more socially acceptable – to acknowledge your miscarriages openly once you have been fully inducted into parenthood, once you reach this point those losses are not supposed to form a part of your present any more, only your past. Any residual grief, trauma, or yearning is supposed to be washed away by the arrival of a longed-for child. After all, you got what you wanted – didn't you? In this way, parenthood makes miscarriage harder to discuss in its full complexity. And by the same stroke, a history of miscarriage can make parenthood harder to discuss fully, too.

When Edward is twelve weeks old, I take him to stay at my mum's for a week. I am exhausted and overwhelmed by my first months as a mother. Pandemic rules and limits on socializing have bounced around since he was born. We have been able to have some visitors, some in-person healthcare, and a few small outings to have a coffee or lunch, but at other points all contact has been cut off, visitors barred from coming inside, cafes and restaurants closed, in-person baby groups halted. Informal childcare has been expressly prohibited by hastily drafted local rules. But now travel restrictions have eased just enough for me to come to Mum's. She cooks for me. She pegs out some of the endless rounds of Edward laundry. She holds him while I shower. She drives us to new places to walk and plans a trip to the beach. She makes me leave the house when I really don't want to, when I don't feel I have the energy, even if it's just for a walk around the block. In these ways, and dozens of others that are barely perceptible, she shows me how life with a baby could be lived and, above all, made to run that bit smoother. Staying with Mum, my edges feel a little less jagged. I realize that this is how you learn to be a mother: from watching other mothers. And this is precisely what I've been missing in lockdown. The realization comes with an echo: this is what is missing in miscarriage, too. Even when we seem saturated with stories of miscarriage – celebrity miscarriage, influencer miscarriage, miscarriage studies on the evening news – it is still rare to hear these stories in real time, or close to it, from the people we know and love. This is perhaps the final frontier in openness. We do not really see miscarriage lived, only reported. We rarely witness someone's reaction and coping process in context, as it happens. A couple might tell us they lost a baby previously, once they are pregnant again or after their child is born. But we do not always see when a friend is cancelling a social event because they are having surgery after a loss, because the pills didn't work, or how much time they took off work afterwards, or whether they choose to commemorate a due date (or not), or what medical treatment and tests they were offered. This is not to say that talking about any of this should be obligatory.

Miscarriage is perhaps an instinctively more private experience than others. All the same, we're often without templates when it happens to us. Just like new mothers kept away from other mothers, we're left with no idea how to actually do this.

A few days into our stay, I hear the news of Chrissy Teigen's miscarriage, via a text from an editor on a newspaper I some-times work for. I look at her message asking if I could write something about it. I stare at the little green bubble of text for a long time. Then I look, briefly, at Teigen's original social media post about losing her son, with its carousel of black and white photos. And I know I cannot do this justice. Not right now. I tell the editor no. Even if I could sit at my laptop for long enough in between feeding Edward, my brain is too slow and waterlogged from weeks of sleeping in two- and three-hour snatches to write coherently. More than that, I do not know how to present my own life and feelings as they stand, not with any degree of hon-esty, clarity, or purpose. I am conscious of my new status as someone who has a baby at home. I am aware of how difficult I used to find reading accounts of miscarriage and pregnancy loss, as told by someone who now has a young family, rather than someone still in the thick of it. But this is not the only reason that the thought of invoking that still-familiar pain of losing babies – too small, too soon – in this particular moment feels almost fraudulent. It is also because I am finding this new life hard. I am struggling to reconcile the reality of parenting with the know-ledge that it is what I have wanted for so long. It is hard to admit that it is hard, let alone that I am actively not enjoying it.

You are uniquely placed, as someone who has tried a reason-ably long time to have a baby, to see the double con society plays on women when it comes to having children: how we are told that attaining motherhood is the most important thing, and yet mothers, when they get there, are treated as the least important thing. You see how grand a pedestal pregnancy is put upon while you are cowering, unseen, in its shadow, but then you also learn how that pedestal is unceremoniously kicked away once your child takes form in the world.

When you are trying to conceive and carry a child without much luck, in a world that continually upholds motherhood as the only moral and meaningful choice for women, you know how being alone in your quiet, tidy house can feel like a rebuke. You know how the small pleasures of unencumbered evenings and weekend lie-ins can sometimes make you feel pointless, even indolent. You know all too well what it is like to sit solo in a coffee shop, surrounded by tables of mums and babies, feeling insignificant next to their prams and changing-bag clobber. You also know that not having children does not mean you are spared all caring responsibilities, financial pressures, or early starts – despite other people's frequent assumptions about how you must live. And yet, when you do manage to have a baby, you also come to know how inadequate postnatal healthcare really is. You now know the physical indignities of new motherhood – leaking, bulging, aching – and just how little time, energy, and support there is to do anything about them. You know how lonely and draining days with no one but a teething, constipated baby can be. You know what it is like to be so tired you are afraid to drive your car; the treacly way your brain and limbs seem to work – or rather, don't. You now know that however hard you and your partner try to parent equally and share the load, the world will thwart you; that the nursery will only ever message you, the mother, about World Book Day costumes; that dads 'babysit' and mums get 'me time' as a substitute for an intact sense of self. You now know that to father a child is a complete sentence, but to mother a child is boundary-less, always ongoing, unfinished, never enough. You also know the constant torn-in-two feeling of craving time away from your child during the day, time to yourself, only to miss them once they are finally asleep, desperate to curl your body around theirs, hungry for the feel of their warm skin.

In short, you've learned first-hand that motherhood is both an 'experience' and an 'institution', as the poet and feminist Adrienne Rich described in her seminal 1986 work *Of Woman Born*. Sitting alongside the actual physical and emotional relationship we have with our children, motherhood is also a social and political construction. Often, what we are encouraged to think of as natural and intrinsic to the maternal experience is really a result of the systems built around it – which 'exonerates men from fatherhood in any authentic sense', traps women into indentured domestic 'servitude', and, above all, aims at ensuring women 'remain under male control'.[1]

I find all the different sides of motherhood equally hard to talk about. In motherland, I am a non-native speaker. On the one hand, I am unwilling to add too much to our pro-natal monoculture, mindful of how much it hurts when you are not part of it, feeling like an increasingly endangered species. For this reason, I hold back from recounting the delicate joys of first smiles and afternoons spent skin-on-skin. I keep to myself the enchantment of seeing flashes of Dan or myself in Edward's emerging features, character, likes, and dislikes. But I also find it hard to join in with others when they vocalize the ways that motherhood is hard. It is hard to admit that the system is letting parents – and especially women – down. I am afraid of seeming to complain; of appearing monstrously ungrateful. So mostly I say nothing. It takes me months to make even a weak joke about my greatest ambition in life being to drink an entire cup of coffee while it's still hot. And still I wince inside as I hear the words leave my mouth.

At the same time, in old support groups, on social media, and with friends with fertility struggles of their own, I am increasingly uncertain of my place; of how much to share. I am conscious that my empathy is no longer a perfect mirror. Once you have a child, you do not immediately forget the sting of pregnancy announcements, the scan photos that barge into your morning via WhatsApp groups, or the online ambush of

Mother's Day. You still get a prickle of envy, and then second-hand anxiety, when someone close to you is pregnant. But you also no longer live with the immense weight of uncertainty as to whether you will ever carry a pregnancy to term. The wondering how that would feel, how I would look heavily pregnant, whether I will get to go through labour, breastfeeding: all of that aching curiosity has been satisfied. I now know what our child looks like, after years of imagining. In *The Time Traveler's Wife*, Audrey Niffenegger's 2003 novel, the protagonist Clare is married to a man who is repeatedly pulled back and forth in time, visiting moments across his past and future, without being able to control when or where he goes. When Clare and Henry decide to start a family, it seems their unborn children share this temporal defect, time-travelling out of Clare's womb and back, ending their brief lives in the process. Three weeks after her fifth miscarriage, Clare is visited by her husband from two years into the future. Breaking their usual rules, he tells her: 'Hang in there. In my present we have a baby.' How many times, in the years before Edward was born, had I wished for a visit from my own benevolent time traveller? Throughout everything, it was the not knowing that I found hardest to live with. So now, I find I censor myself in both conversations about parenting and conversations about pregnancy loss. What I long for, but can scarcely find, are conversations about how it feels when these two things become meshed – messily – together.

There is also relatively little published science that would help me to make sense of this current chapter of my life. In fact, as researchers writing in the *Lancet* in 2021 pointed out, the longer-term consequences of miscarriage, especially repeated miscarriage, is perhaps the greatest unknown of all, in a field full of unasked and unanswered questions. There are hints, though. Both depression and anxiety triggered by pregnancy loss can persist 'well past' the arrival of a healthy baby, a 2011 study published in the *British Journal of Psychiatry* found, for example. In fact, the study authors concluded there was no evidence at all that a living child improved anxiety and depression symptoms, both of which were common in women who'd had either a miscarriage or a stillbirth, and which often overlapped. For this study, researchers used data from around 13,000 women living in England who answered questionnaires about their mental health during pregnancy and then at four points after birth, starting when their babies were eight weeks old and finishing when their children were nearly three. Dr Emma Robertson Blackmore, a psychiatrist and the study's lead author, said at the time: 'Our study clearly shows that the birth of a healthy baby does not resolve the mental health problems that many women experience after a miscarriage or stillbirth.'[2] This, to me, seems hugely significant, and directly contradicts the pervasive perception that having a baby after previous pregnancy loss must be an unmitigated explosion of happiness – a healing miracle, an answer to all your prayers.

More recent research, too, has pointed to a history of miscarriage being a predictor for postnatal depression. For example, a review of existing studies published in 2021, which attempted to identify the greatest risk factors for postnatal depression during the Covid-19 pandemic, listed miscarriage as one of its key predictive categories for depressive symptoms after giving birth.[3] And a Chinese study, from 2018, suggested that previous experiences of miscarriage increased the risk of suicidal thoughts in the early post-partum period.[4] Back in 2011, Dr Robertson Blackmore pointed out: 'When assessing if a woman is at risk of antenatal or postnatal depression, previous pregnancy loss is usually not taken into account in the same way as other risk factors such as a family history of depression, stressful life events or a lack of social support.' And this remains true more than ten years on. Perinatal mental health has, quite rightly, been made more of a priority in the UK in recent years. Postnatal depression is thought to affect more than one in ten.

Suicide is still the leading pregnancy-related cause of death within a year of giving birth. Postnatal anxiety, which may cause insomnia and panic attacks, is less well recognized – both by the general public and by healthcare professionals – but is still common. Women are now supposed to be asked basic screening questions about their mental health at their first appointment in pregnancy and at the six-week postnatal check-up they are meant to have with their GP. Yet guidance to healthcare professionals on spotting perinatal mental health problems and intervening early does not flag previous pregnancy loss as a possible contributing factor to be aware of. Unlike other considerations, doctors are not encouraged to ask about it.[5] Certainly, no one – not my GP, nor my health visitor, and none of the midwives – raised the subject with me directly after Edward was born. But it is unlikely to be something women raise voluntarily. There is immense psychological and social pressure on all new mothers to 'enjoy every minute' (a hyperbolic standard we apply to few other life experiences). But it takes on a particular, tormenting resonance if there is also an internal pressure, knowing what it took to get here, knowing the pain of being earlier denied these precious minutes of motherhood. *You must be so happy . . . Is it everything you hoped it would be?* How could you ever admit that the answer was anything but an emphatic, straightforward 'yes'?

A history of miscarriage may also have health consequences long after your fertile years have passed. The review of the available evidence on miscarriage published in the *Lancet* in 2021 pointed out that there seems to be a risk of both cardiovascular disease and blood clots later in life for women who've had recurrent miscarriage.* What's not yet known is *why* two or more

---

* In fact, a report published in the *European Heart Journal*, also in 2021, recommended that, due to an apparent link between heart disease later in life and a history of miscarriage, it should be considered important medical information for

miscarriages should increase your risk of heart disease and blood clots later in life. It's been suggested that there could be overlapping risk factors for miscarriages and for cardiovascular disease – smoking, obesity, alcohol consumption - but cardiac experts have also pointed out that there could be an underlying causal link, with both recurrent pregnancy loss and future cardiovascular events happening due to some form of endothelial dysfunction (how blood vessels behave).[6] Remember how one in six heart attacks in people under fifty has been found to be caused by the condition antiphospholipid syndrome – which is also a common cause of recurrent miscarriage? How many more heart attacks might we be able to prevent if we not only knew more about miscarriage as a potential early-warning sign, but also didn't treat pregnancy loss as largely irrelevant once someone has had their family?

I run into the legacy of my miscarriages again and again in motherhood. Like at the very beginning, when Edward is losing more weight than is considered normal for newborns, but no one is quite sure why. Despite appearing to latch on and feed well, despite scoring positively on various questionnaires and breastfeeding charts, his weight continues to fall. Everyone has different, conflicting advice for me. One midwife says I should top up with formula. Another says I absolutely must *not* top up with formula; what I need to do is to pump extra milk after every feed to boost my supply. Knowing that this kind of difficulty in the early days of breastfeeding is relatively normal does not help. In fact, it's not really the feeding issue itself that bothers me. What panics me is that no one can point to a reason for what is happening. Despite the number on the scales, he

---

cardiac doctors to ask about. 'Pregnancy history should be an integral part of cardiovascular risk assessment,' suggested the report, which summarized the views of an international panel of experts. (See note 6.)

seems perfectly healthy, he *seems* to be feeding fine. It's unexplainable. And the prospect of there being some hidden problem with my body – or Edward's – that medics cannot discover or define shatters the glass around some internal alarm.

Sometimes, my former self taps me on the shoulder when my parenting reality differs from the widely proclaimed norm. Before we got out of hospital, more than one person had warned us, in a jovial sort of a way, that the first night home with your first baby is the longest night of your life. And yet, the wild anxiety never arrived as promised. That first night, time passed evenly and just as I expected it should. For the first time in weeks, maybe even months, the minutes didn't stretch out or dart about. Reflecting on this the next morning, I wasn't at all surprised; after all, the terror and weight of trying to keep a baby alive were not exactly new to me and Dan. Besides, after pregnancy, it has been a pleasant surprise to discover just how much information there is to turn to when it comes to baby care once they're actually born. There is so much more data you can collect, so many signs you can monitor, and so many more places you can go to for help. Have they had enough wet nappies today? How frequently have they fed? What colour are their hands and feet? You can gently pinch their skin to check for warnings of dehydration. You can lie in bed and listen to them breathing. Of course, while this all feels like an unexpected bonus, it also reconfirms how little information we had to sustain us before. It feels a little like performing a high-wire stunt without a harness and realizing only afterwards that safety equipment *is* available.

Another occasion I tend to collide with my past self is on especially difficult parenting days, inspiring intense guilt. Maternal ambivalence is a taboo that is being slowly chipped away: the idea that motherhood is not fulfilling all the time is one that barely seems radical any more. Yet I still find it hard to own up to. Nearly forty years ago, Adrienne Rich described perfectly the emotional tug of war that so many who care for small children will still recognize today: 'I could love so much better, I told myself, after even a quarter-hour of selfishness, of peace, of detachment from my children. A few minutes! But it was as if an invisible thread would pull taut between us and break, to the child's sense of inconsolable abandonment, if I moved – not even physically, but in spirit – into a realm beyond our tightly circumscribed life together.' Guilt is an emotion almost taken for granted in motherhood now – it is not unique to women who have struggled to get here. Rich describes how turning her attention from her child sometimes felt 'as if my placenta had begun to refuse him oxygen'.[7] I recognize this sensation. And it threatens to transmogrify guilt into something monstrous, when your placenta has literally failed before – or, at least, that's what you suspect might have happened.

Even the joyful experiences of motherhood are not always free from reminders, triggers, unresolved grief. When you have only had miscarriages, you suspect, but do not know first-hand, just how stark the difference is between having a baby and losing one. Bringing Edward home confirmed it. With every card, gift, or text from a colleague I'd not heard from in years, with every eager question about his name or his weight, with every request for a photo, and with every milestone passed, there was also a shiver of retroactive loss and loneliness. The thought would arrive, like a cloud passing over the sun: *Oh, so this is what we've been missing, all this time.*

Unfortunately, as it stands, there is little room in our current institution of motherhood to examine much or any of this. How could there be when there are so many other fires to fight? When only 15 per cent of women get the dedicated appointment with their GP they are supposed to have after having a baby. When pelvic floor dysfunction and how to treat it is not consistently included in training for GPs, nurses, and midwives. When 30,000 women every year are left traumatized by their labour experience – and when life-limiting, incontinence-causing injuries from giving birth may affect as many as one in ten. When too many workplaces treat mothers as a burden to be offloaded as quickly – and cheaply – as possible. When childcare is inadequately and patchily subsidized. When school holiday days vastly outnumber the days of annual leave most employees get. When we seem to have tacitly agreed, to paraphrase the MP Stella Creasy, that motherhood should be a struggle,* it's not hard to see how miscarriage falls off the agenda once people become parents. Which is not the same as it ceasing to matter.

At the same time, there may be a parallel set of limitations on talking about miscarriage for those who do not go on to have children. This, too, is likely both self-imposed and externally enforced. Those who are childless not by choice live under a dual burden of exclusion and misunderstanding. First, they're affected by the social stigma that attaches to *all* people who do not have children. They are excluded from popular narratives around 'hard-working families'. They are decried as selfish by religious leaders. In a world still struggling to treat people without children as fully equal, valuable members of society, talking about the specifics of why you do not have children is made more difficult. Against such a backdrop, it is not hard to see how you might fear playing into unhelpful ideas and stereotypes about 'good' childless people (tragic but tolerated) and 'bad' childless people (feckless, self-involved – to be disapproved of). Laid over the top of this is widespread cultural insensitivity and

* Creasy, who has spoken about her own experience of miscarriage, put it like this in a newspaper interview in 2022: 'People say motherhood has to be a struggle and a juggle – when did we agree that? When did we go, "Yeah, this basic thing that humanity has to do to keep existing, we're going to make it really hard – just for 50 per cent of people [mothers]. The other 50 per cent [fathers] we're going to give them a gold medal if they appear with their baby because they're caring and modern."' (Stella Creasy: 'When did we agree motherhood had to be a struggle?', *Sunday Times*, 16 January 2022.)

a failure to truly understand that, sometimes, people try very hard to have children and it just does not happen for them. If this is you, to continue talking about your miscarriages, or to push for improvement in this area of medicine, is to continue to acknowledge something openly that many are uncomfortable with: that there was something you wanted from life, but didn't get. Quite apart from the high emotional price of retelling the details of what may amount to an irreconcilable grief, even if people do wish to tell this side of the story, are we prepared to hear it? As a society, we are practically allergic to the narrative that, try as you might, things didn't work out. In conversations around fertility and trying for a family, people reinforce a belief that where there is a will, there is a way. And yet, you cannot 'just adopt'. It's not true that 'there's always IVF'. Above all, deciding to stop trying is not 'giving up'. Studies have repeatedly shown that prospective fertility patients overestimate the success rates of IVF. Estimates vary, but it could be that as many as 30 per cent of people who have more than three miscarriages in a row do not go on to have living children. But where are the human stories behind this side of the statistics? And if there is very little research into being a parent after pregnancy loss, there is next to nothing about those who never get there. Specialist nurse and researcher Dr Sarah Bailey knows through her work running a recurrent-miscarriage clinic that, for some, while there may be no definitive reason they can't conceive or carry a child, they reach a point at which the thought of enduring another pregnancy simply becomes untenable. Whether this moment comes after five losses, six losses, or more than ten, will vary with individuals, she says. Yet no research into this experience has been undertaken.

And, of course, miscarriage can happen after you've already had children – though this, too, is an under-recognized strand of the story. Once you have one child, the problem of your fertility, if it was ever in question, is presumed to have been

resolved, in perpetuity. Despite Edward's arrival, I have no way
of knowing if any subsequent pregnancies will end in yet more
miscarriages. There is no more certainty on that front for us
than there was two years ago. We can only guess at whether the
progesterone made the difference this time, or whether it was
luck – and, therefore, whether we will get that lucky again.
Many other people have miscarriages even when they previously only had uncomplicated pregnancies and healthy children.
Likewise, secondary infertility – being unable to conceive after
you've had one child without issue or intervention – is thought
to be at least as common as primary infertility, affecting around
one in eight couples. Given that the risk of miscarriage rises
with age, due to the increased likelihood of lethal chromosomal
defects, it is logical to assume that for a lot of women their first
encounter with miscarriage will come once they've had other
children. If anything, this should be the miscarriage story we
are most used to hearing. Yet, on the whole, we are less sympathetic to this scenario. We try to ignore it, as though it were less
important. People are told that 'at least' they have one child. Or
'be grateful for the kids you do have', as if expressing a desire
for another, or grief for one that didn't make it, is axiomatically
to dishonour your other children. And so this group, too, are
shamed into silence. It means that while we've normalized
discussing family size as though it were always a straightforward choice – like ordering from a menu: *two girls and a boy,
with a side of twins, please* – we rarely hear from those whose
reproductive lives go out on a slow fade, letting go of the idea
of another family member gradually, bit by bit, until someone
says 'enough, no more', after one loss, or one negative test, too
many.

All of this helps to explain why miscarriage remains only
partially understood: as a subject, it perpetually loses its campaigning constituency. Whichever way your reproductive fate
unfolds, you come to feel that there is a statute of limitations

on your sadness; on talking about it. But this doesn't mean you forget.

It's October when I get home from Mum's. We're immediately thrown back into a local lockdown. I spend long days on my own with Edward, as, unlike the first lockdown, Dan is no longer working from home. I walk for miles every day, with Edward in a sling, partly because there is nothing else to do, and partly because it is often the only way he will sleep. Feeling his curled, prawn body against mine, the solid fact of his skull against my breastbone, never stops being a rush: a flood of oxytocin and dopamine, love and happiness. But sometimes, quite often, I do feel like I'm being tested. Just when my world has expanded in one way, everything else has been stripped out of it. As if this were the sly genie's parting shot. 'What?' it seems to smirk. 'You said *all* you wanted was a baby.'

Mostly, I try hard not to think about the things we are not getting to do, the people we are not getting to see, except when I need to remind myself of why it feels hard. On those days, I can't help listing what is missing: all the things that would make looking after Edward a bit easier; all the things I could do to escape the house and feel a bit more myself. I hold these things in my mind: the baby groups, the coffee mornings, the swimming pool, the hairdresser, the trips to Granny's or Nana's, the dinners out with a willing babysitter – I roll them around, using them like prayer beads, trying to keep my mind from wandering. *Lockdown is why this is hard. Lockdown is why I'm not always enjoying it.* I need to keep my thoughts trained this way, because otherwise I will notice the low-down, dirty fear I have that my unhappiness stems from the fact that I was simply not meant to be a mother. After all, hadn't my body given me enough hints? There is another nagging feeling I'm trying to squash. So many of the things I now long for, that gave my life meaning and texture, were fully available to me when I was trying to conceive,

yet I often treated them as though they were nothing. I resent
this creeping impression that the grass really is always greener.
Or perhaps what I resent is how miscarriage numbed me to so
much that was good in my life.

Day follows day follows interminable day. Just before
Edward reaches six months old – his half-birthday – I start to
write again, just for the short, random snatches of time he gives
me during his first nap of the day, when I am least tired. Sometimes I get an hour. Sometimes I get ten minutes. It does not
escape me that it is the same coping mechanism I used after my
miscarriages. Nothing changes, not immediately. Motherhood
continues to be hard. Motherhood continues to be magical.
Sometimes it is both in the space of a single afternoon, a single
hour. I am more fulfilled in this primal role than I have ever
been. And sometimes I am still empty. Yet somewhere along
the way, in the depths of winter, something starts to shift. The
storm has not blown over, but there is a slight change in the
atmospheric pressure that seems to signal to me that it *will* pass.
So motherhood was not going to bring about the instant and
complete sense of belonging I had perhaps assumed. Neither is
it going to make up for all that had gone before. With each
passing week, I find it easier to accept that I cannot go back. I
also see that I will not get this time again. Slowly, slowly, there
is a lesson that is unfurling – something about life and how
happiness works. But just when I think I have grasped it, when
I try to set it out in my mind or put it into words, it flits away
again – like a bird taking flight upon catching your eye.

Epilogue

'Everything happens for a reason'

(January 2021 – six months old)

'Home is where one starts from. As we grow older
The world becomes stranger, the pattern more complicated
Of dead and living.'

T. S. Eliot, 'East Coker', from *Four Quartets*

My son's bedroom is painted a buttery yellow. If you were to mix this colour on an artist's palette, you would start with lemony lead-tin yellow and add just a dab of mushroom-grey to keep it from being sickly. It is a colour that makes me think of Cotswolds stone, Norfolk sand, and wild primroses. It is my favourite room in the house. It has warm, oak floorboards and a candy-striped blind I had specially made to fit inside the awkward window, which has a chunk of rough-hewn rock for a lintel. Edward doesn't actually sleep in here yet, but it is still full of him, somehow. Just thinking of standing inside his room is like being warmed by the sun. It is beautiful. It is also not the nursery I once assumed I would decorate. No. That room was going to be dove grey: 'Polished Pebble'. That room belongs to a different house, a different life.

The temptation with a story like this one is to conclude that it was always meant to happen this way. That 'everything happens for a reason'. When well-meaning people say this to me now, I put on the same too-tight smile that I'd wear when similar platitudes were offered to me after each miscarriage. *'It was probably for the best'* . . . *'It wasn't meant to be'* . . . *'This baby just wasn't part of life's plan for you'*. There is a term for these kinds of expressions, coined by the psychiatrist Robert Jay Lifton: they are 'thought-terminating clichés'. They act as a roadblock to critical thinking or to probing further in a way that would lead to meaningful understanding. As Lifton wrote, 'the most far-reaching and complex of human problems are compressed into brief, highly reductive, definitive-sounding phrases, easily memorized and easily expressed'. We reach for thought-terminating clichés a lot in conversations around pregnancy loss and infertility, and all they do is let us off the hook. If we comfort ourselves that it was always meant to work out like this, then there is no need to think about it any longer. In thinking and talking this way, we also extinguish any urgency when it comes to finding ways to prevent miscarriage, to make pregnancy safer, or to improve IVF success rates.

Somehow, even in secular societies, we haven't quite shaken off an impression that to try to bring fertility more within our control is an insult to some higher power – that this whole area is something we, as mere mortals, would do well not to meddle with. But to expand and extend our knowledge of the very beginnings of human biology is no more playing God or defying a preordained cosmic order than developing vaccines or ensuring we have clean water to drink. Really, it is hubris in the extreme to imagine that by mastering the intricacies and inner workings of sperm, ovum, the uterine immune system, DNA, and RNA we would somehow be assuming total control of our fate in a way that would make us less human.

I do not, personally, believe in a god. But I do believe in the enormous, unconquerable power of chance. Chance has been fucking with us all our lives. No medical advances, no level of scientific knowledge could ever hope to overcome this. Dan and I met a long time before this story started. But we almost didn't. He had been directing the university pantomime, which I auditioned for (badly). I almost stayed home that night, as I had a cold. Years later, Dan would tell me how he almost missed out on joining the pantomime society in the first place. He'd auditioned as a new student, but rather than go for a drink in the union bar with the others afterwards, he'd decided to go home. After waiting an unusually long time for a bus on Manchester's Oxford Road, he convinced himself to go back and be sociable. He met his best friend that night – the best man at our wedding. He also discovered his contact details had been written down wrong on the sign-up sheet. Had the bus come sooner, he might have assumed he hadn't got a part and simply got on with a different life.

We could play this game for ever. What about the near misses of our parents? Our grandparents? Dan's grandmother – now Edward's Oma – escaped to England from Nazi Germany on the Kindertransport. That the shape and trajectory of our lives rests on so much and so little is impossible to fully comprehend. Perhaps it is the essential magic of being alive. Being able to control when sperm meets egg, or to be able to make a pregnancy stick, does not threaten this.

Of course, having said all this, I do feel like it was always meant to be Edward. As much as it sounds like another thought-terminating cliché, I cannot imagine my life another way. It's not the case that I don't remember what life was like before him, but it is true that it feels as though he has always been here. It's complicated.

Here, then, is one final reason miscarriage wants for status and examination, and why it can become harder, not easier, to talk about. There is a certain amount of cognitive dissonance that arises through both wanting the child you have, who might not otherwise have arrived, and still wishing you had not lost previous pregnancies. On the one hand, you feel this is the child you were always meant to have. It was always going to be them. You know this in your marrow. You feel it in the nucleus of every cell and in the hairs that prickle on the back of your neck. But that is not exactly the same as being glad that it happened this way and not the other way. It is not reducible to 'everything happens for a reason'. I want Edward. I also wish I hadn't miscarried before. I want both things; both versions of my life. But to try to explain this risks being misunderstood and in potentially very hurtful ways. It risks being mistaken for an absolutely prohibited admission: maternal regret. This is perhaps our deepest social taboo – and with good reason. It is a terrible thing to make a child feel unwanted. This, of course, is not what your feelings about a previous loss actually mean. Not even slightly. Still, it is easier to simply stop talking rather than trespass on this forbidden territory, even accidentally.

It defies both logic and biology, this predicament. I want to have met the child I carried four years ago, and the three after that. I also want Edward. My love for him is my deepest anchor. It is my oxygen and my gravity. On one of the many long afternoons at home with him in lockdown, I hear an unfamiliar word on a radio show that stops me in my tracks: 'bathybic'. It means, the speaker explains, 'relating to the deepest parts of the sea'. This, I think, is what my love for Edward is like. Sometimes I feel ashamed that I could still yearn for anything else, however abstract, however impossible.

The way my mind tries to square this circle – when I feel wistful and sad and then guilty – is by conceptualizing the baby I could have had back then as Edward's older sibling, though I know deep down that isn't really how it works; I know one thing always leads to another, then another. On and on. So sometimes, my brain plays a different kind of trick. Sometimes, it tells me that Edward and the baby we didn't have four years ago are one and the same. It is not a different life altogether that I am missing; it is that I could have been living this one four years earlier.

It is an unremarkable morning in January when Dad phones to tell me that my grandma has died. I'm distracted and in the middle of putting away some washing.

'Hello! Everything all right?' I say, not really expecting that it isn't.

And then his voice cracks and I freeze.

The day is unmade. I speak to my brother on the phone. We both say how much we wish we could all be together as a family. But that is not allowed at the moment. Among the many things I think and feel, in the hours after I learn she is gone, is a quiet anger that Edward has missed her by four years. He could have known her for four years, had he only been born then instead of now. I know, even as I notice myself thinking it, that this is not rational.

But perhaps this is what I really believe. A friend I made not long after my fourth miscarriage told me how in her faith it's believed that the souls of babies lost in pregnancy come back to you, reincarnated in your subsequent children. Normally, I recoiled when people encouraged me to consider my miscarriages through the framework of their own religious views. But not this time. I wasn't sure that I really believed in a soul in any literal sense, yet I couldn't help being comforted by the idea; even more so, when, on a different day, I find out that embryos shed cells into a mother's bloodstream, which can then remain in circulation in her blood and tissue for years after pregnancy, a phenomenon known as microchimerism. So perhaps, somehow, some tiny part of my previous pregnancies has made its way into Edward after all. Then again, perhaps this, too, is an attempt to tie up loose ends in a way that makes the ineffable that bit easier to understand.

And I am wary of burdening Edward with too much meaning, when he should be allowed simply to belong to himself. I do not wish for him to live with the label of 'miracle baby'. *'The one who stayed'* . . . *'The boy who lived'*. However well intentioned this might be, he should not have to grow up in the shadow of putative children. Instead, what I want most for him is the simple freedom of an unfreighted, ordinary existence, secure in his place in the world, secure in our love. That is far more special than any mythology we could hope to construct for him.

Unable to do anything else, after hearing about Grandma, Dan and I go for a walk, taking our usual loop. My hands curl protectively around the front of Edward's body, strapped to me in his carrier. He is big enough now to face outwards, and his hands and feet wave and jiggle as I walk. Dan and I stroll mostly in silence, but it is comfortable silence. Life for us is better than it has ever been, with our baby, in the home we chose, in a place that feels like we could put down roots. It is also worse, as of this morning. Things have not worked out perfectly after all, but then they were never going to.

We walk for thirty minutes until we are almost back where we started. We turn off the main road and on to our lane. If this were a film, a thin trail of smoke would be curling from our chimney, beckoning us home. But there is no fire in the stove – yet. Later, there will be. Later, there will also be fish and chips. And a glass of red wine. Much later, there will be daffodils in the verge along the lane again. And after that, bluebells, which in turn will give way to cow parsley and the tall, purple spikes of willowherb. Later still, we will be able to take Edward to visit his whole family. We will also take him on holiday, holding him upright in the sand and the waves. We will watch him transform from a timid lockdown baby, who cries if a passing dogwalker says hello, into a little entertainer who cranes his neck in cafes, seeking out anyone who might be susceptible to his charm. Later — and at last — we will dance at my brother's wedding and raise a glass to absent friends. To Grandma. Not long after that, I will realize I no longer feel I'm play-acting the role of mother; I am simply living it. I will go into my son's room in the morning, he will flash me a toothy grin and shout ''Ello, Mama!', followed swiftly by a demand for 'Brep-fast!'

But for now, Dan and I have nowhere else to go and nowhere else to be. There is only one way from here, and we pick our steps carefully on the shingled track that leads to our house. At dusk, it looks like a dark river, snaking down the hill. Even more so for being slick with snowmelt from the fields. We follow it. We follow it back to where our extraordinary, ordinary life awaits.

Further Reading

J. Bueno, *The Brink of Being: Talking About Miscarriage* (London, Virago, 2019)

L. Enright, *Vagina: A Re-Education* (London, Allen & Unwin, 2020)

K. Figes, *Life After Birth* (London, Penguin, 2000)

N. Gaskin, *Life After Baby Loss: A Companion and Guide for Parents* (London, Vermilion, 2018)

O. Gordon, *The First Breath: How Modern Medicine Saves the Most Fragile Lives* (London, Bluebird, 2019)

E. Haslett and G. Griffith, *Big Fat Negative: The Essential Guide to Infertility, IVF and the Trials of Trying for a Baby* (London, Piatkus, 2022)

A. Kimball, *The Seed: Infertility Is a Feminist Issue* (Toronto, Coach House Books, 2019)

L. Regan, *Miscarriage: What Every Woman Needs to Know* (London, Orion Spring, 2018)

J. Zucker, *I Had a Miscarriage: A Memoir, A Movement* (New York, Feminist Press at the City University of New York, 2021)

Resources

Charities/websites

Tommy's
https://www.tommys.org

The Miscarriage Association
https://www.miscarriageassociation.org.uk

The Ectopic Pregnancy Trust
https://ectopic.org.uk

Arc Antenatal Results and Choices
https://www.arc-uk.org

Cradle
https://cradlecharity.org

Sands
https://www.sands.org.uk

Petals
https://petalscharity.org

BPAS (British Pregnancy Advisory Service)
https://www.bpas.org

Pregnant Then Screwed
https://pregnantthenscrewed.com

Five X More
https://fivexmore.com

Gateway Women
https://gateway-women.com

Podcasts

The Big Fat Negative
https://podcasts.apple.com/gb/podcast/big-fat-negative-ttc-
fertility-infertility-and-ivf/id1431698726

Fertility Life Raft
https://podcasts.apple.com/gb/podcast/fertility-life-raft/
id1436164035

Finally Pregnant
https://podcasts.apple.com/gb/podcast/finally-pregnant/
id1463544731

Time To Talk TFMR
https://talktfmr.podbean.com/

The Worst Girl Gang Ever
https://podcasts.apple.com/gb/podcast/the-worst-girl-gang-
ever/id1524031149

Notes

Introduction

1 E. Webber, Twitter (now deleted), as reported in N. Burton, 'Want to "call out" Chrissy Teigen over her pregnancy loss and her pro-choice views? Read this first', *Independent*, 5 October 2020: https://www.independent.co.uk/voices/chrissy-teigen-john-legend-miscarriage-baby-pregnancy-instagram-abortion-anti-choice-b742546.html [accessed 11 June 2022]

2 C. M. McCarthy et al., 'The general populations' understanding of first trimester miscarriage: a cross sectional survey', *European Journal of Obstetrics & Gynecology and Reproductive Biology*, 254 (2020), 200–205: https://pubmed.ncbi.nlm.nih.gov/33010694/ [accessed 13 May 2022]

3 '#MisCourage', Tommy's: https://www.tommys.org/get-involved/campaigns/miscourage [accessed 13 May 2022]

4 B. O'Neill, 'Do we really need to know about Meghan Markle's miscarriage?', Spiked, 26 November 2020: https://www.spiked-online.com/2020/11/26/do-we-really-need-to-know-about-meghan-markles-miscarriage/ [accessed 21 July 2022]

5 C. Long, 'Can we stop all the woe-is-me over our wombs? We're women, not victims', *Sunday Times*, 29 November 2020: https://www.thetimes.co.uk/article/can-we-stop-all-the-woe-is-me-over-our-wombs-were-women-not-victims-tcghnf2mk [accessed 21 July 2022]

6 M. Obama, 'Becoming Michelle: a First Lady's journey with Robin Roberts', ABC, 12 November 2018: https://abc.com/shows/2020/episode-guide/2018-11/11-becoming-michelle-a-first-ladys-journey-with-robin-roberts [accessed 8 July 2022]

1 'It's so common'

1 J. Bueno, *The Brink of Being: Talking About Miscarriage* (London, Virago, 2019)

2 L. Regan, *Miscarriage: What Every Woman Needs to Know* (London, Orion Spring, 2018)

3 World Health Organization, 'Why we need to talk about losing a baby': https://www.who.int/news-room/spotlight/why-we-need-to-talk-about-losing-a-baby [accessed 31 January 2021]

4 S. Quenby et al., 'Miscarriage matters: the epidemiological, physical, psychological, and economic costs of early pregnancy loss', *Lancet*, 397:10285 (2021), 1658–67:

https://www.thelancet.com/journals/lancet/article/PIIS0140-6736(21)00682-6/full-text [accessed 13 May 2022]

5 MBRACE-UK, 'Saving lives, improving mothers' care: lessons learned to inform maternity care from the UK and Ireland Confidential Enquiries into Maternal Deaths and Morbidity 2017–19', November 2021: https://www.npeu.ox.ac.uk/assets/downloads/mbrrace-uk/reports/maternal-report-2021/MBRRACE-UK_Maternal_Report_2021_-_FINAL_-_WEB_VERSION.pdf [accessed 13 May 2022]

6 MBRRACE-UK, 'Perinatal Mortality Surveillance Report: Summary', 2018: https://www.npeu.ox.ac.uk/assets/downloads/mbrrace-uk/reports/perinatal-surveillance-report-2018/MBRRACE-UK_Perinatal_Surveillance_Report_2018_-_summary.pdf [accessed 13 May 2022]

7 J. Jardine et al., 'Adverse pregnancy outcomes attributable to socioeconomic and ethnic inequalities in England: a national cohort study', *Lancet*, 398:10314 (2021), 1905–12: https://www.thelancet.com/journals/lancet/article/PIIS0140-6736(21)01595-6/fulltext [accessed 13 May 2022]

8 S. Quenby et al., 'Miscarriage matters', op. cit.

2 'At least it was early'

1 University of Leeds, 'Human heart development slower than other mammals', 21 February 2013: https://www.leeds.ac.uk/news-health/news/article/3368/human-heart-development-slower-than-other-mammals [accessed 13 May 2022]

2 K. Doka, *Disenfranchised Grief* (Massachusetts, Lexington Books, 1989)

3 C. Murray Parkes and H. G. Prigerson, *Bereavement: Studies of Grief in Adult Life*, 4th edn (London, Penguin, 2010)

4 N. S. Macklon et al., 'Conception to ongoing pregnancy: the "black box" of early pregnancy loss', *Human Reproduction Update*, 8:4 (2002), 333–43: https://pubmed.ncbi.nlm.nih.gov/12206468/ [accessed 13 May 2022]

5 Ibid.

6 R. Martin, 'Meiotic errors in human oogenesis and spermatogenesis', *Reproductive BioMedicine Online*, 16:4 (2008), 523–31 https://www.rbmojournal.com/article/S1472-6483(10)60459-2/pdf

7 K. Niakan et al., 'Human pre-implantation embryo development', *Development*, 139:5 (2012), 829–41: https://www.ncbi.nlm.nih.gov/pmc/articles/PMC3274351/ [accessed 13 May 2022]

8 S. Han, 'The chemical pregnancy: technology, mothering, and the making of a reproductive experience', *Journal of the Motherhood Initiative for Research and Community Involvement*, 5:2 (2015): https://jarm.journals.yorku.ca/index.php/jarm/article/view/39759 [accessed 13 May 2022]

9 Quoted in J. M. W. Slack, *From Egg to Embryo: Determinative Events in Early Development* (Cambridge University Press, 1983), p. 1

10 G. Janes, 'Early stage of human embryo development seen for the first time', BioNews, 1122, 19 November 2021: https://www.bionews.org.uk/page_160595 [accessed 16 May 2022]

11 Quoted in S. Reardon, 'Human embryos grown in lab for longer than ever before', *Nature*, 4 May 2016: https://www.nature.com/articles/533015a [accessed 11 June 2022]

12 K. Chaudhry et al., 'Anembryonic pregnancy', StatPearls, 5 February 2022: https://www.ncbi.nlm.nih.gov/books/NBK499938/ [accessed 16 May 2022]

13 L. Regan, *Miscarriage: What Every Woman Needs to Know* (London, Orion Spring, 2018), p. 17

3 'It's just nature's way'

1 S. Quenby et al., 'Miscarriage matters: the epidemiological, physical, psychological, and economic costs of early pregnancy loss', *Lancet*, 397:10285 (2021), 1658–67: https://www.thelancet.com/journals/lancet/article/PIIS0140-6736(21)00682-6/fulltext [accessed 13 May 2022]

2 'Coping with a Miscarriage', Miscarriage Association leaflet, April 1987, Wellcome Collection

3 L. Regan, *Miscarriage: What Every Woman Needs to Know* (London, Orion Spring, 2018), p. 61; L. Regan et al., 'Influence of past reproductive performance on risk of spontaneous abortion', *BMJ*, 299:6698 (1989), 541–5: https://www.bmj.com/content/299/6698/541 [accessed 16 May 2022]

4 A. Coomarasamy et al., 'A randomized trial of progesterone in women with bleeding in early pregnancy', *New England Journal of Medicine*, 380 (2019), 1815–24: https://www.nejm.org/doi/full/10.1056/NEJMoa1813730 [accessed 16 May 2022]

4 'It's probably nothing'

1 L. Regan, *Miscarriage: What Every Woman Needs to Know* (London, Orion Spring, 2018), p. 14

2 'Premature birth statistics', Tommy's: https://www.tommys.org/pregnancy-information/premature-birth/premature-birth-statistics [accessed 16 May 2022]

3 R. N. Pillai et al., 'Role of serum biomarkers in the prediction of outcome in women with threatened miscarriage: a systematic review and diagnostic accuracy meta-analysis', *Human Reproduction Update*, 22:2 (2016), 228–39: https://academic.oup.com/humupd/article/22/2/228/2457894 [accessed 18 May 2022]

4 M. G. Tuuli et al., 'Perinatal outcomes in women with subchorionic hematoma: a systematic review and meta-analysis', *Obstetrics & Gynecology*, 117:5 (2011), 1205–12: https://pubmed.ncbi.nlm.nih.gov/21508763/ [accessed 17 May 2022]

5 K. L. Anderson et al., 'Outcomes of in vitro fertilization pregnancies complicated by subchorionic hematoma detected on first-trimester ultrasound', *F&S Reports*, 1:2 (2020), 149–53: https://www.sciencedirect.com/science/article/pii/S2666334120300192#bib1

6 L. Detti et al., 'Early pregnancy ultrasound measurements and prediction of first trimester pregnancy loss: a logistic model', *Scientific Reports*, 10:1545 (2020): https://www.nature.com/articles/s41598-020-58114-3 [accessed 17 May 2022]

7 St Mary's Hospital Emergency Gynaecology Unit, 'Bleeding in Early Pregnancy (Threatened Miscarriage)': https://mft.nhs.uk/app/uploads/sites/4/2018/04/02-81-Bleeding-in-early-pregnancy-threatened-miscarriage-June-2018.pdf [accessed 30 June 2022]

8 Geisinger, 'Bleeding in early pregnancy: when should you worry?', Geisinger, 12 May 2021: https://www.geisinger.org/health-and-wellness/wellness-articles/2019/08/21/18/35/bleeding-in-early-pregnancy-when-should-you-worry [accessed 17 May 2022]

9 H. Murkoff, *What to Expect When You're Expecting*, 5th edn (London, Simon & Schuster, 2016), p. 140

10 R. Elliot, 'The Meanings of Miscarriage in Twentieth-Century Britain', in *Navigating Miscarriage: Social, Medical and Conceptual Perspectives*, ed. S. Kilshaw and K. Borg (New York and Oxford, Berghahn, 2020), p. 167

11 R. H. F. van Oppenraaij et al., 'Predicting adverse obstetric outcome after early pregnancy events and complications: a review', *Human Reproduction Update*, 15:4 (2009): https://academic.oup.com/humupd/article/15/4/409/733496 [accessed 17 May 2022]

12 R. Hasan et al., 'Association between first-trimester vaginal bleeding and miscarriage', *Obstetrics & Gynecology*, 114:4 (2009), 860–67: https://www.ncbi.nlm.nih.gov/pmc/articles/PMC2828396/ [accessed 17 May 2022]

13 Ibid.

5 'She doesn't carry well'

1 S. Kilshaw and K. Borg (eds), *Navigating Miscarriage: Social, Medical and Conceptual Perspectives* (New York and Oxford, Berghahn, 2020), p. 39.

2 S. Quenby et al., 'Miscarriage matters: the epidemiological, physical, psychological, and economic costs of early pregnancy loss', *Lancet*, 397:10285 (2021), 1658–67: https://www.thelancet.com/journals/lancet/article/PIIS0140-6736(21)00682-6/fulltext [accessed 13 May 2022]

3 L. Regan, *Miscarriage: What Every Woman Needs to Know* (London, Orion Spring, 2018), p. 65

4 N. A. du Fossé et al., 'Advanced paternal age is associated with an increased risk of spontaneous miscarriage: a systematic review and meta-analysis', *Human*

Reproduction Update, 26:5 (2020), 650–69: https://academic.oup.com/humupd/article/26/5/650/5827629 [accessed 17 May 2022]

5 M. C. Magnus et al., 'Role of maternal age and pregnancy history in risk of miscarriage: prospective register based study', *BMJ*, 364:1869 (2019): https://www.bmj.com/content/364/bmj.l869 [accessed 17 May 2022]

6 '17 years old', Miscarriage Association: https://www.miscarriageassociation.org.uk/story/17-years-old/ [accessed 17 May 2022]

7 S. Quenby et al., 'Miscarriage matters', op. cit.

8 W. Lo et al., 'The effect of body mass index on the outcome of pregnancy in women with recurrent miscarriage', *Journal of Family & Community Medicine*, 19:3 (2012), 167–71: https://www.ncbi.nlm.nih.gov/pmc/articles/PMC3515955/ [accessed 17 May 2022]

9 I. V. Landres, 'Karyotype of miscarriages in relation to maternal weight', *Human Reproduction*, 25:5 (2010), 1123–6: https://pubmed.ncbi.nlm.nih.gov/20190263/ [accessed 17 May 2022]

10 A. M. Clark et al., 'Weight loss in obese infertile women results in improvement in reproductive outcome for all forms of fertility treatment', *Human Reproduction*, 13:6 (1998), 1502–5: https://pubmed.ncbi.nlm.nih.gov/9688382/ [accessed 17 May 2022]

11 A. M. F. Woolner et al., 'Family history and risk of miscarriage: a systematic review and meta-analysis of observational studies', *Acta Obstericia et Gynaecologica Scandinavica*, 99:12 (2020), 1584–94: https://obgyn.onlinelibrary.wiley.com/doi/full/10.1111/aogs.13940 [accessed 17 May 2022]

12 L. Regan, op. cit., pp. 205–7

6 'In case something happens'

1 A. Boss et al., 'Placental formation in early pregnancy: how is the centre of the placenta made?', *Human Reproduction Update*, 24:6 (2018), 750–60: https://academic.oup.com/humupd/article/24/6/750/5102231 [accessed 17 May 2020]

2 S. Mukherjee et al., 'Risk of miscarriage among black women and white women in a US prospective cohort study', *American Journal of Epidemiology*, 177:11 (2013), 1271–8: https://academic.oup.com/aje/article/177/11/1271/97504 [accessed 18 May 2022]

3 J. Olszynko-Gryn, 'The feminist appropriation of pregnancy testing in 1970s Britain', *Women's History Review*, 28:6 (2017), 869–94: https://www.ncbi.nlm.nih.gov/pmc/articles/PMC6817328/ [accessed 18 May 2022]

4 L. Freidenfelds, *The Myth of the Perfect Pregnancy: A History of Miscarriage in America* (Oxford University Press, 2020), p. 26

5 S. Withycombe, *Lost: Miscarriage in Nineteenth Century America* (Rutgers University Press, 2018), p. 48

6 T. Harpel and J. Hertzog, ' "I thought my heart would burst": the role of ultrasound technology on expectant grandmotherhood', *Journal of Family Issues*,

October 2009: https://journals.sagepub.com/doi/abs/10.1177/0192513X09348491 [accessed 18 May 2022]

7 S. Withycombe, *Lost*, op. cit., p. 15

8 A. Andrew et al., 'Women much more likely than men to give up paid work or cut hours after childbirth even when they earn more', Institute for Fiscal Studies, 12 March 2021: https://ifs.org.uk/publications/15359 [accessed 18 May 2022]

9 Equality and Human Rights Commission, 'Employers in the dark ages over recruitment of pregnant women and new mothers', 19 February 2018: https://www.equalityhumanrights.com/en/our-work/news/employers-dark-ages-over-recruitment-pregnant-women-and-new-mothers [accessed 18 May 2022]

10 '40% of managers avoid hiring younger women to get around maternity leave', *Guardian*, 12 August 2014: https://www.theguardian.com/money/2014/aug/12/managers-avoid-hiring-younger-women-maternity-leave [accessed 18 May 2022]

11 'Miscarriage, stillbirth and neonatal death – rights to time off and pay', Maternity Action, March 2022: https://maternityaction.org.uk/advice/miscarriage-stillbirth-and-neonatal-death-rights-to-time-off-and-pay-for-parents/ [accessed 18 May 2022]

12 S. Kilshaw, 'God's design, thwarted plans: women's experience of miscarriage in Qatar and England' in *Navigating Miscarriage: Social, Medical and Conceptual Perspectives*, ed. S. Kilshaw and K. Borg (New York and Oxford, Berghahn, 2020), p. 339

7 'Products of conception'

1 'A review of support available for loss in early and late pregnancy', NHS Improving Quality, February 2014: https://www.england.nhs.uk/improvement-hub/wp-content/uploads/sites/44/2017/11/Available-Support-for-Pregnancy-Loss.pdf [accessed 18 May 2022]

2 M. S. Fejzo et al., 'Placenta and appetite genes GDF15 and IGFBP7 are associated with hyperemesis gravidarum', *Nature Communications*, 9:1176 (2018): https://www.ncbi.nlm.nih.gov/pmc/articles/PMC5862842/ [accessed 19 May 2022]

3 Y. Yang et al., 'Circulating fibroblast growth factor 21 as a potential biomarker for missed abortion in humans', *Fertility and Sterility*, 116:4 (2021), 1040–49: https://www.fertstert.org/article/S0015-0282(21)00473-8/pdf [accessed 19 May 2022]

8 'It can't be helped'

1 A. Coomarasamy et al., 'Recurrent miscarriage: evidence to accelerate action', *Lancet*, 397:10285 (2021), 1675–82: https://www.thelancet.com/journals/lancet/article/PIIS0140-6736(21)00681-4/fulltext [accessed 19 May 2022]

2 According to obstetrician Stuart Campbell, quoted in O. Gordon, *The First Breath: How Modern Medicine Saves the Most Fragile Lives* (London, Bluebird, 2019), p. 68

3 L. Zhang et al., 'Gender biases in estimation of others' pain', *Journal of Pain*, 22:9 (2021), 1048–59: https://www.sciencedaily.com/releases/2021/04/210406164124.htm

4 C. M. Borkhoff et al., 'Patient gender affects the referral and recommendation for total joint arthroplasty', *Clinical Orthopaedics and Related Research*, 469:7 (2011), 1829–37: https://pubmed.ncbi.nlm.nih.gov/21448775/ [accessed 19 May 2022]

5 A. A. Mirin et al., 'Research update: the relation between ME/CFS disease burden and research funding in the USA', *Work*, 66:2 (2020), 277–82: https://pubmed.ncbi.nlm.nih.gov/32568148/#:~:text=Results%3A%20We%20find%20the%20disease,that%20commensurate%20with%20disease%20burden

6 UK Clinical Research Collaboration, 'UK Health Research Analysis 2018', Medical Research Council, 2020: https://hrcsonline.net/wp-content/uploads/2020/01/UK-Health-Research-Analysis-2018-for-web-v1-28Jan2020.pdf [accessed 19 May 2022]

7 S. Moalem, *The Better Half: On the Genetic Superiority of Women* (London, Allen Lane, 2020), p. 178

8 S. Guthrie et al., 'Understanding pregnancy research needs and priorities in the UK', RAND Europe: https://www.rand.org/randeurope/research/projects/uk-pregnancy-research-needs.html [accessed 19 May 2022]

9 S. Tewary et al., 'Impact of sitagliptin on endometrial mesenchymal stem-like progenitor cells: a randomised, double-blind placebo-controlled feasibility trial', *EBioMedicine*, 51:102597 (2020): https://www.thelancet.com/journals/ebiom/article/PIIS2352-3964(19)30812-6/fulltext [accessed 19 May 2022]

10 M. Al-Biate, 'Effect of metformin on early pregnancy loss in women with polycystic ovary syndrome', *Taiwanese Journal of Obstetrics and Gynecology*, 54:3 (2015), 266–9: https://pubmed.ncbi.nlm.nih.gov/26166338/ [accessed 29 June 2022]

11 A. Coomarasamy et al., 'Recurrent miscarriage', op. cit.

12 G. I. Swyer and D. Daley, 'Progesterone implantation in habitual abortion', *British Medical Journal*, 1:4819 (1953), 1073–7: https://www.ncbi.nlm.nih.gov/pmc/articles/PMC2016475/?page=1 [accessed 19 May 2022]

13 A. Coomarasamy et al., 'A randomized trial of progesterone in women with recurrent miscarriages', *New England Journal of Medicine*, 373 (2015), 2141–8: https://www.nejm.org/doi/full/10.1056/NEJMoa1504927?query=featured_home [accessed 19 May 2022]

14 D. M. Haas et al., 'Progestogen for preventing miscarriage in women with recurrent miscarriage of unclear etiology', *Cochrane Database of Systematic Reviews*, October 2018: https://www.cochranelibrary.com/cdsr/doi/10.1002/14651858.CD003511.pub4/full [accessed 19 May 2022]

15 M. Al-Memar et al., 'The association between vaginal bacterial composition and miscarriage: a nested case-control study', *British Journal of Obstetrics and Gynaecology*, 127:2 (2020), 264–74: https://pubmed.ncbi.nlm.nih.gov/31573753/ [accessed 19 May 2022]

16 K. Grewal et al., 'O-129 *Lactobacillus* deplete vaginal microbial composition is associated with chromosomally normal miscarriage and local inflammation', *Human*

Reproduction, 36:S1 (2021): https://academic.oup.com/humrep/article-abstract/36/ Supplement_1/deab126.054/6344065 [accessed 19 May 2022]

17 C. Ober et al., 'Mononuclear-cell immunisation in prevention of recurrent miscarriages: a randomised trial', *Lancet*, 354:9176 (1999), 365–9: https://pubmed.ncbi. nlm.nih.gov/10437864/ [accessed 19 May 2022]

18 D. Jarrett, *33 Meditations on Death* (London, Doubleday, 2020), p. 114

9 'It's not a real baby yet'

1 A. Gottlieb, *The Afterlife is Where We Come From: The Culture of Infancy in West Africa* (University of Chicago Press, 2004), p. 41

2 L. Freidenfelds, *The Myth of the Perfect Pregnancy: A History of Miscarriage in America* (Oxford University Press, 2020), p. 14

3 A. Gottlieb, 'Do infants have religion? The spiritual lives of Beng babies', *American Anthropologist*, 100:1 (1998), 122–35

4 'A Guide for the Jewish Parent on Miscarriages, Stillbirths & Neonatal Death', United Synagogue: https://www.theus.org.uk/sites/default/files/still%20birth%20singles.pdf

5 B. P. Fallon and G. B. Mychaliska, 'Development of an artificial placenta for support of premature infants: narrative review of the history, recent milestones, and future innovation', *Translational Pediatrics*, 10:5 (2021), 1470–85: https://pubmed.ncbi.nlm.nih.gov/34189106/ [accessed 20 May 2022]

6 'Senate Joint Resolution 314: a joint resolution designating October 1988 as "Pregnancy and Infant Loss Awareness Month"', 100th Congress (1987–88), October 1988: https://www.congress.gov/bill/100th-congress/senate-joint-resolution/314 [accessed 20 May 2022]

7 L. J. Reagan, 'From hazard to blessing to tragedy: representations of miscarriage in twentieth-century America', *Feminist Studies*, 29:2 (2003), 356–78: https:// www.jstor.org/stable/3178514?read-now=1&seq=7 [accessed 23 May 2022]

8 R. Elliot, 'The Meanings of Miscarriage in Twentieth-Century Britain', in *Navigating Miscarriage: Social, Medical and Conceptual Perspectives*, ed. S. Kilshaw and K. Borg (New York and Oxford, Berghahn, 2020), pp. 171–2

9 L. Brown, J. Brown and S. Freeman, *Our Miracle Called Louise: A Parents' Story* (London, Paddington Press, 1979), p. 118

10 K. Dow, 'Now she's just an ordinary baby: the birth of IVF in the British press', *Sociology*, 53:2 (2019), 314–29: https://journals.sagepub.com/doi/full/10.1177/ 0038038518757953 [accessed 20 May 2022]

11 A. Kimball, *The Seed: Infertility is a Feminist Issue* (Toronto, Coach House Books, 2019), p. 66

12 A. Kimball, 'Unpregnant: the silent, secret grief of miscarriage', *Globe and Mail*, 3 December 2015: https://www.theglobeandmail.com/life/parenting/unpregnant-the-silent-secret-grief-of-miscarriage/article27576775/ [accessed 20 June 2022]

13 'Press release – Significant pro-life victory: attempt to introduce extreme changes to abortion law fails', Right To Life, November 2021: https://righttolife.org.uk/news/press-release-significant-pro-life-victory-attempt-to-introduce-extreme-changes-to-abortion-law-fails

10 'Better safe than sorry'

1 A. Brown, *Covid Babies: How Pandemic Health Measures Undermined Pregnancy, Birth and Early Parenting* (London, Pinter & Martin, 2021), pp. 50–57

2 J. Agg, 'Anguish of the stillbirth dilemma', *Daily Mail*, 11 October 2021: https://www.dailymail.co.uk/health/article-10081521/Anguish-stillbirth-dilemma-Dramatic-proposal-NICE-save-infant-lives.html [accessed 20 May 2022]

3 A. Khalil et al., 'Change in obstetric attendance and activities during the Covid-19 pandemic', *Lancet Infectious Diseases*, 21:5 (2021), e115: https://www.sciencedirect.com/science/article/pii/S1473309920307799 [accessed 20 May 2022]

4 R. Elliot, 'The Meanings of Miscarriage in Twentieth-Century Britain', in *Navigating Miscarriage: Social, Medical & Conceptual Perspectives*, ed. S. Kilshaw and K. Borg (New York and Oxford, Berghahn, 2020), p. 172

5 'Test is said to cut miscarriage peril', *New York Times*, 16 April 1958: https://timesmachine.nytimes.com/timesmachine/1958/04/16/83409089.html?pageNumber=25 [accessed 22 May 2022]

6 W. J. Dieckmann et al., 'Does the administration of diethylstilbestrol during pregnancy have therapeutic value?', *American Journal of Obstetrics & Gynecology*, 66:6 (1953), 1062–81: https://pubmed.ncbi.nlm.nih.gov/13104505/ [accessed 23 May 2022]

7 M. Knight et al., 'Include pregnant women in research – particularly covid-19 research', *BMJ*, 370:m3305 (2020): https://www.bmj.com/content/370/bmj.m3305?ijkey=1a067392cfd50ae6de505f9e9fd672aac3972c6b&keytype2=tf_ipsecsha [accessed 23 May 2022]

8 R. Schraer, 'Covid vaccine: fertility and miscarriage claims fact-checked', BBC, 11 August 2021: https://www.bbc.co.uk/news/health-57552527 [accessed 23 May 2022]

11 'Women's stuff'

1 C. N. Jayasena et al., 'Reduced testicular steroidogenesis and increased semen oxidative stress in male partners as novel markers of recurrent miscarriage', *Clinical Chemistry*, 65:1 (2019), 161–9: https://academic.oup.com/clinchem/article/65/1/161/5607916 [accessed 23 May 2022]

2 K. A. Turner et al., 'Male infertility is a women's health issue – research and clinical evaluation of male infertility is needed', *Cells*, 9:4 (2020), 990: https://www.

ncbi.nlm.nih.gov/pmc/articles/PMC7226946/#B17-cells-09-00990 [accessed 23 May 2022]

3 C. Barratt et al., "Man up": the importance and strategy for placing male reproductive health centre stage in the political and research agenda', *Human Reproduction*, 33:4 (2018), 541–5: https://www.ncbi.nlm.nih.gov/pmc/articles/PMC5989613/ [accessed 23 May 2022]

4 K. A. Turner et al., 'Male infertility is a women's health issue', op. cit.

5 H. Levine et al., 'Temporal trends in sperm count: a systematic review and meta-regression analysis', *Human Reproductive Update*, 23:6 (2017), 646–59: https://pubmed.ncbi.nlm.nih.gov/28981654/ [accessed 23 May 2022]

6 K. A. Turner et al., 'Male infertility is a women's health issue', op. cit.

7 R. Ramasamy et al., 'Fluorescence in situ hybridization detects increased sperm aneuploidy in men with recurrent pregnancy loss', *Fertility and Sterility*, 103:4 (2015), 906–9: https://pubmed.ncbi.nlm.nih.gov/25707335/ [accessed 23 May 2022]

8 N. A. du Fossé et al., 'Paternal smoking is associated with an increased risk of pregnancy loss in a dose-dependent manner: a systematic review and meta-analysis', *F&S Reviews*, 2:3 (2021), 227–38: https://www.sciencedirect.com/science/article/pii/S2666571921000128 [accessed 23 May 2022]

9 L. Regan, *Miscarriage: What Every Woman Needs to Know* (London, Orion Spring, 2018), p. 64

10 A. Moscrop, 'Can sex during pregnancy cause a miscarriage? A concise history of not knowing', *British Journal of General Practice*, 62:597 (2012), e308–10: https://www.ncbi.nlm.nih.gov/pmc/articles/PMC3310038/ [accessed 23 May 2022]

11 J. R. Fisher and K. Hammarberg, 'Psychological and social aspects of infertility in men: an overview of the evidence and implications for psychologically informed clinical care and future research', *Asian Journal of Andrology*, 14:1 (2012), 121–9: https://www.ncbi.nlm.nih.gov/pmc/articles/PMC3735147/ [accessed 23 May 2022]

12 C. Due et al., 'The impact of pregnancy loss on men's health and wellbeing: a systematic review', *BMC Pregnancy Childbirth*, 17:380 (2017): https://bmcpregnancychildbirth.biomedcentral.com/articles/10.1186/s12884-017-1560-9 [accessed 23 May 2022]

13 D. Wojnar, 'Miscarriage experiences of lesbian couples', *Journal of Midwifery & Women's Health*, 52:5 (2007), 479–85: https://pubmed.ncbi.nlm.nih.gov/17826711/ [accessed 23 May 2022]

14 E. Peel, 'Pregnancy loss in lesbian and bisexual women: an online survey of experiences', *Human Reproduction*, 25:3 (2010), 721–7: https://www.ncbi.nlm.nih.gov/pmc/articles/PMC2817567/#DEP441C43 [accessed 23 May 2022]

15 D. W. Riggs et al., 'Gay men's experiences of surrogacy clinics in India', *Journal of Family Planning and Reproductive Health Care*, 41:1 (2014), 48–53: https://pubmed.ncbi.nlm.nih.gov/25351689/ [accessed 23 May 2022]; I. Ziv and Y. Freund-Eschar,

'The pregnancy experience of gay couples expecting a child through overseas surrogacy', *Family Journal*, 23:2 (2014): https://journals.sagepub.com/doi/abs/10.1177/1066480714565107 [accessed 23 May 2022]

16 H. Williams et al., 'Men living through multiple miscarriages: protocol for a qualitative exploration of experiences and support requirements', *BMJ Open*, 10:5, (2020), e035967: https://bmjopen.bmj.com/content/10/5/e035967 [accessed 23 May 2022]

17 J. R. Fisher and K. Hammarberg, 'Psychological and social aspects of infertility in men', op. cit.

18 'How climate change could be causing miscarriages in Bangladesh', BBC, 26 November 2018: https://www.bbc.co.uk/news/world-asia-45715550 [accessed 23 May 2022]

12 'Just stay positive'

1 H. D. L Ockhuijsen et al., 'Coping after recurrent miscarriage: uncertainty and bracing for the worst', *Journal of Family Planning and Reproductive Health Care*, 39:4 (2013), 260–66: https://pubmed.ncbi.nlm.nih.gov/23329740/ [accessed 23 May 2022]

2 S. Bailey et al., 'Effective support following recurrent pregnancy loss: a randomized controlled feasibility and acceptability study', *Reproductive Biomedicine Online*, 40:5 (2020), 729–42: https://pubmed.ncbi.nlm.nih.gov/32444166/ [accessed 23 May 2022]

3 C. Hanson, *A Cultural History of Pregnancy: Pregnancy, Medicine and Culture, 1750–2000* (London, Palgrave Macmillan, 2004), p. 28

4 L. J. Reagan, 'From hazard to blessing to tragedy: representations of miscarriage in twentieth-century America', *Feminist Studies*, 29:2 (2003), 356–78: https://www.jstor.org/stable/3178514?read-now=1&seq=7 [accessed 23 May 2022]

5 J. Schaffir, 'Do patients associate adverse pregnancy outcomes with folkloric beliefs?', *Archives of Women's Mental Health*, 10:6 (2007), 301–4: https://pubmed.ncbi.nlm.nih.gov/17710367/ [accessed 23 May 2022], as cited in F. Qu et al., 'The association between psychological stress and miscarriage: a systematic review and meta-analysis', *Scientific Reports*, 7:1731 (2017): https://www.ncbi.nlm.nih.gov/pmc/articles/PMC5431920/#CR41 [accessed 23 May 2022]

6 J. Nynas et al., 'Depression and anxiety following early pregnancy loss: recommendations for primary care providers', *Primary Care Companion for CNS Disorders*, 17:1 (2015): https://www.ncbi.nlm.nih.gov/pmc/articles/PMC4468887/ [accessed 23 May 2022]

7 J. Farren et al., 'Post-traumatic stress, anxiety and depression following miscarriage or ectopic pregnancy: a prospective cohort study', *BMJ Open*, 6:11 (2016), e011864: https://pubmed.ncbi.nlm.nih.gov/27807081/ [accessed 23 May 2022]

8 I. H. Lok et al., 'A 1-year longitudinal study of psychological morbidity after miscarriage', *Fertility and Sterility*, 93:6 (2010), 1966–75: https://www.fertstert.org/article/S0015-0282(08)04743-2/pdf [accessed 23 May 2022]

13 'They'll come when they're ready'

1 A. M. Jukic et al., 'Length of human pregnancy and contributors to its natural variation', *Human Reproduction*, 28:10 (2013), 2848–55: https://academic.oup.com/humrep/article/28/10/2848/620772?login=true [accessed 23 May 2022]

2 G. Wightman Lawson, 'Naegele's rule and the length of pregnancy – a review', *ANZJOG*, 61:2 (2021), 177–82: https://obgyn.onlinelibrary.wiley.com/doi/full/10.1111/ajo.13253] [accessed 23 May 2022]

3 A. S. Oberg et al., 'Maternal and fetal genetic contributions to postterm birth: familial clustering in a population-based sample of 475,429 Swedish births', *American Journal of Epidemiology*, 177:6 (2013), 531–7: https://academic.oup.com/aje/article/177/6/531/160108 [accessed 23 May 2022]

4 E. Digitale, 'Stanford researchers identify blood markers that indicate labor is approaching', *Stanford Medicine,* 5 May 2021: https://med.stanford.edu/news/all-news/2021/05/blood-markers-indicate-labor-approaching.html [accessed 24 May 2020]

5 P. Middleton et al., 'Induction of labour at or beyond 37 weeks' gestation', *Cochrane Database of Systematic Reviews*, 7:7 (2020): https://www.cochranelibrary.com/cdsr/doi/10.1002/14651858.CD004945.pub5/full [accessed 24 May 2022]

6 H. G. Dahlen et al., 'Intrapartum interventions and outcomes for women and children following induction of labour at term in uncomplicated pregnancies: a 16-year population-based linked data study', *BMJ Open*, 11:6 (2021), e047040: https://bmjopen.bmj.com/content/11/6/e047040 [accessed 24 May 2022]

7 A. E. P. Heazell et al., 'Association between maternal sleep practices and late stillbirth – findings from a stillbirth case-control study', *British Journal of Obstetrics and Gynaeology*, 125:2 (2018), 254–62: https://doi.org/10.1111/1471-0528.14967 [accessed 24 May 2022]

8 A. A. Moraitis et al., 'Fetal umbilical artery Doppler as a tool for universal third trimester screening: a systematic review and meta-analysis of diagnostic test accuracy', *Placenta*, 108 (2021), 47–54: https://pubmed.ncbi.nlm.nih.gov/33819861/ [accessed 24 May 2022]; L. Al-Hafez et al., 'Routine third-trimester ultrasound in low-risk pregnancies and perinatal death: a systematic review and meta-analysis', *American Journal of Obstetrics & Gynecology*, 2:4 (2020), 100242: https://pubmed.ncbi.nlm.nih.gov/33345941/ [accessed 24 May 2022]; J. E. Norman et al., 'Awareness of fetal movements and care package to reduce fetal mortality (AFFIRM): a stepped-wedge, cluster-randomised trial', *Lancet*, 392:10158 (2018), 1629–38: https://www.thelancet.com/journals/lancet/article/PIIS0140-6736(18)31543-5/fulltext#seccestitle80 [accessed 24 May 2022]

9 Z. Sultana et al., 'Is there a role for placental senescence in the genesis of obstetric complications and fetal growth restriction?', *American Journal of Obstetrics & Gynecology*, 218:2 (2018), S762–73: https://www.ajog.org/article/S0002-9378(17)32332-3/fulltext [accessed 24 May 2022]

10 B. C. Baker et al., 'Sexually dimorphic patterns in maternal circulating micro-RNAs in pregnancies complicated by fetal growth restriction', *Biology of Sex Differences*, 12:61 (2021): https://pubmed.ncbi.nlm.nih.gov/34789323/ [accessed 24 May 2022]; L. Armstrong-Buisseret et al., 'Standard care informed by the result of a placental growth factor blood test versus standard care alone in women with reduced fetal movement at or after 36+0 weeks' gestation: a pilot randomised controlled trial', *Pilot and Feasibility Studies*, 6:23 (2020): https://pilotfeasibilitystudies.biomedcentral.com/articles/10.1186/s40814-020-0561-z [accessed 24 May 2022]

11 S. Quenby et al., 'Miscarriage matters', op. cit.

12 J. Sandall et al., 'Midwife-led continuity models versus other models of care for childbearing women', *Cochrane Database of Systematic Reviews*, 4:4 (2016): https://www.cochranelibrary.com/cdsr/doi/10.1002/14651858.CD004667.pub5/full [accessed 24 May 2022]

14 'Enjoy every minute'

1 A. Rich, *Of Woman Born: Motherhood as Experience and Institution* (London, W. W. Norton, 1986), pp. 13–14

2 E. Robertson Blackmore et al., 'Previous prenatal loss as a predictor of perinatal depression and anxiety', *British Journal of Psychiatry*, May 2011: https://pubmed.ncbi.nlm.nih.gov/21372060/

3 S. Usmani et al., 'Risk factors for postpartum depression during Covid-19 pandemic: a systematic literature review', *Journal of Primary Care & Community Health*, 12 (2021), 1–9 https://journals.sagepub.com/doi/10.1177/21501327211059348?url_ver=Z39.88-2003&rfr_id=ori%3Arid%3Acrossref.org&rfr_dat=cr_pub++0pubmed& [accessed 25 May 2022]

4 P. Shi et al., 'Maternal depression and suicide at immediate prenatal and early postpartum periods and psychosocial risk factors', *Psychiatry Research*, 261 (2018), 298–306: https://www.sciencedirect.com/science/article/abs/pii/S0165178116318881?via%3Dihub [accessed 25 May 2022]

5 'Recognising mental health problems in pregnancy and the postnatal period and referral', in Clinical Guideline CG192, NICE, 11 February 2020: https://www.nice.org.uk/guidance/cg192/chapter/1-Recommendations#recognising-mental-health-problems-in-pregnancy-and-the-postnatal-period-and-referral-2 [accessed 25 Marcy 2022]

6 A. Maas et al., 'Cardiovascular health after menopause transition, pregnancy disorders, and other gynaecologic conditions: a consensus document from European cardiologists, gynaecologists, and endocrinologists', *European Heart Journal*, 42:10 (2021), 967–84: https://pubmed.ncbi.nlm.nih.gov/33495787/ [accessed June 2022]

7 A. Rich, *Of Woman Born*, op. cit., p. 23

Acknowledgements

First and foremost, if you are reading this because you have found yourself facing similar terrain on your way to having a family, I sincerely hope that what I've written here has been a comfort. Please also know that I wish you had never felt the need for this book in the first place. This book started life as a blog. Along the way, I have sometimes been asked if writing about our experiences has been therapeutic, and the honest answer to that (understandable) question is: not exactly. The therapeutic part has been hearing from so many others who have experienced something similar. To everyone who has ever sent me a kind message on social media, commented on a blog post, or poured difficult feelings into a heartfelt email – I cannot thank you enough.

There are many people who gave up their precious time to talk to me in the name of research for this book. To every single one of you, thank you for sharing your work and your wisdom so generously. I am especially grateful to those who have trusted me to include their personal stories in these pages. I hope I have done you – and your babies – justice.

To the team at Tommy's, for all that you do: thank you for trying to answer the questions that so many seem to think aren't worth asking. Thank you, too, to Jane Fisher at ARC and to Ruth Bender-Atik of the Miscarriage Association for your sound advice and words of encouragement.

I am indebted to the incredible team at Transworld for making this idea an ink-and-paper reality. But in particular, thank you to my brilliant editors Zoe Berville and Helena Gonda for caring so deeply about this book and its message; to Kate Fox for steering the ship; to Alex Newby for copy-editing; and to Beci Kelly for the beautiful cover design.

This book might not have come into being without the opportunity to write parts of my story in articles for newspapers and magazines. For that, I am grateful to Josephine Forster, Clare Longrigg, Emma Rowley, Sarah Tomczak and Natasha Lunn. There is one Fleet Street editor I must thank in particular, however, and that is the inimitable Justine Hancock, who not only commissioned the first piece I wrote on the subject of pregnancy loss, shortly after my first miscarriage, but who also had the – possibly unenviable – task of coaching me through writing my first newspaper feature ever (I won't say how long ago that was). This book would not exist were it not for everything you have taught me.

Thank you to everyone at The Soho Agency, not least to Julian Alexander for the flash of title inspiration, and especially to my wonderful agent Niamh O'Grady, for spotting that there was a book here and for being the cheerleader I so often need.

Thank you to my earliest readers, Polly Glass and Hayley Manning. Thanks also to Libby Galvin – editorial support takes many forms, including gossip, walks, coffees, pad thai, and Psycle classes. And thank you to Heather Tulloch for Zoom wine and for listening to me for the last twenty-five years (yes, I had to get the calculator out – and no, I can't believe it, either).

Mum, I hope you know you are the hero of this story.

To Jo, who I wish was still here to read this.

To Edward, for making me a mother.

Finally, there is one other person I need to thank, who I could never thank enough. First, for living through all of this with me and then for supporting our family in a thousand different ways as I tried to commit it to paper. For Dan, for everything.

Jennie Agg is an acclaimed health and science journalist, whose work has appeared in *The Times*, *Guardian*, *Mail*, *Telegraph*, *Red*, *Grazia* and *Women's Health*. She is the author of the award-winning blog *The Uterus Monologues*, through which she has charted her own experience of recurrent miscarriage as well as helping other women to share their stories of infertility and pregnancy loss.